Living with Cancer

THE YEAR WHEN EVEN THE DOG GOT CANCER

The story of how one family continues to live with cancer

By

Jan Caston

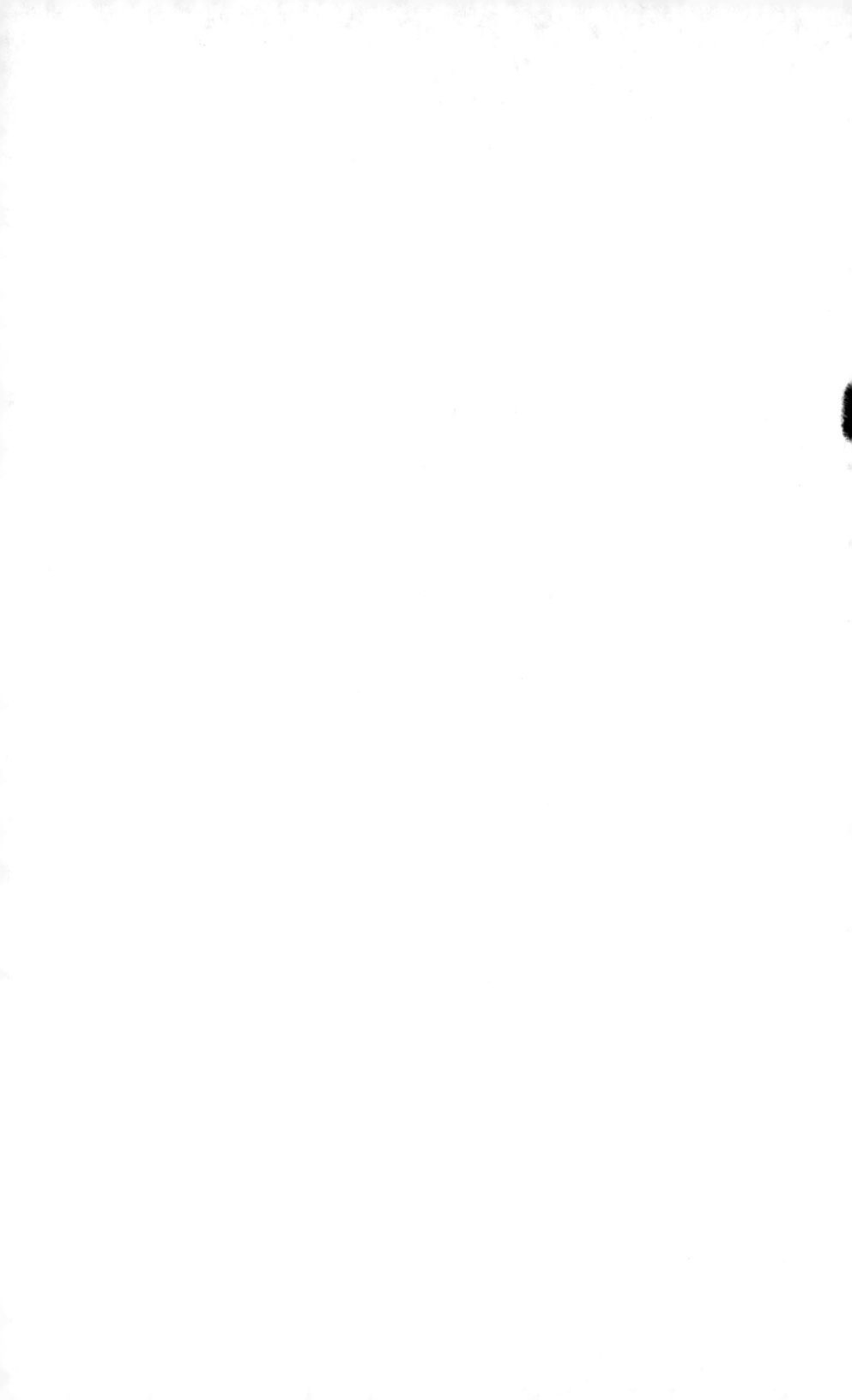

INTRODUCTION

Many books and articles have been written about cancer. Most concentrate on the courage of cancer patients. Not so much has been written about living with cancer long term and the effect it has on families.

Living with Cancer - The Year When Even the Dog Got Cancer follows one family as it deals with four different cases of cancer at the same time over one year. Written from the perspective of the carer who can only watch and help, it aims to give hope and confidence to those living with cancer that this frightening illness can be survived and that life can go on.

Jan Caston is a Writer for the Screen and Stage. Her husband, George, has lived with cancer for over ten years. In 2012, her mother, good friend and even the family dog received treatment for cancer too.

This is the story of how one family dealt with the problems and stress cancer brings and still had fun whilst doing it.

All profits from the sale of this book will be donated to further the work of the Oncology and Nephrology teams at Jersey General Hospital, Jersey, Channel Islands, Great Britain.

Published and Distributed by Amazon.com 2013

ISBN13 978-1484108970

For George,

Mum,

Bonnie

and Bonzo

who always make me smile.

CONTENTS:

INTRODUCTION

CHAPTER ONE

Cancer! Why Him? Why Us?

CHAPTER TWO

Three Out Of Four People In The UK Get Cancer

CHAPTER THREE

2012 – One Hell Of A Year For Olympians

CHAPTER FOUR

Ajay and A.J. – Always Two Of Everything!

CHAPTER FIVE

Keeping Going When Everything Is Falling Apart

CHAPTER SIX

The Absolute Pits: Part One

CHAPTER SEVEN

The Absolute Pits: Part Two

CHAPTER EIGHT

Hopes And Desires

CHAPTER NINE

Preparing For The Inevitable

CHAPTER TEN

And -Again!- We Get On With Living With Cancer

EPILOGUE

CHAPTER ONE

Cancer! Why Him? Why Us?

Quite simply, there is no answer to either of those questions. For my family, to even start getting the questions into perspective, you have to go back many years and the story has to start with a different illness, not cancer.

As I start to write this book on the first day of January 2013 I am ever conscious that another anniversary is about to happen in five days' time. This anniversary is far more important for our family than just any old New Year with its firework frenzy of celebrations. It's an anniversary we quietly, and with great gratitude, celebrate every year, not only for our own family, but also for the family we have never met who made it all possible.

On 6th January 1997 my beloved husband, George, received the gift of a kidney transplant from the UK National Organ Donor Register. And that kidney is still going strong today.

We celebrate that kidney's arrival in our family every year just the same as we'd celebrate the arrival of a child. The transplanted kidney is twenty years younger than George and we look after it as if it is a baby.

George got the call at 5pm on Friday 5th January 1997. I was in our sitting room with my Mum and Dad lazily watching the animated film, A Hundred and One Dalmatians, when the phone rang. George went to answer it. My eyes stayed on the television but my ears honed in to George in the hall answering what seemed like a weird set of bizarre questions.

"Yes. I'm feeling very well, thank you."

"No. I haven't had any chest infection."

"It depends if I can get a plane."

"We've been snowed in here for four days. The airport might still be closed."

I rushed through to join George.

"Is that the call?" I mouthed as he wrote down a load of instructions.

THE CALL! The one from the Transplant Co-Ordinator we were prepared for but had been warned might never come.

He nodded, grim faced.

I read what he was scribbling down. St Mary's, Portsmouth. Meon 5 - Transplant Ward. He turned the paper towards me as he underlined, "Must be there by 9.30 tonight!"

What happened next took place in that flurry of activity which, whilst it's happening, seems to be going in slow motion.

As I threw things into suitcases, George contacted the on-call co-ordinator at Jersey Hospital who got us both on a flight departing forty five minutes later to Southampton. It was the first flight that had been able to leave the Island of Jersey, where we live, for four days. The unexpected snow was beautiful, but the ice and fog that went with it brought the Island to a grinding halt. Snow still lay a foot deep on either side of roads gritted with sand from the seashore. We raced our brand new 4x4 to the airport, parked it haphazardly and ran in. Mum would have to arrange for a friend to pick it up the next day because neither she nor Dad was confident enough to drive such a big car. At that point, we couldn't care less if we ever saw the car again.

"Are you the transplant?" A Flybe representative was waiting for us with boarding cards. "You've got ten minutes to get to the gate. You're in luck. We've had to hold the plane for a head injury that needs to get to hospital in Southampton."

Luck! I remember even then thinking sadly, "How awful that our piece of luck comes from someone else's sorrow."

If you are a member of a family who receives a transplant, you never forget what a gift of life a transplant is; but you also never forget that it came as a result of someone else's death – someone else's bad luck. So, I've long treated luck with healthy scepticism.

As they rushed us through security, I forgot to pick up my handbag with identification, money, contact details; everything we'd need in England. An older man raced after me to give it me back. "He's had The Call ..." I tried to explain. "We know. Good luck. And run."

Speeding through Jersey Airport it was as if word had already gone around and everyone knew why two dishevelled people were hurtling through their midst. "Good lucks" followed us as we showed boarding cards, crashed through an already empty departure lounge and sped up the steps to the plane.

We were shown to the back two seats in the cabin and apart from saying "thank you" to the Stewardess who strapped us in we could do nothing on the thirty minute flight but clutch each other's hands in awe struck silence. The seconds to 9.30 p.m. were ticking away far too rapidly.

George had already been told that he was the seventh person they'd contacted that day for that particular kidney. The six other people who were possible matches in the UK they'd contacted before him all had chest infections. They weren't fit enough to have so big an operation. Its partner kidney was going to be airlifted to a patient in Sheffield, the only other match identified in the UK. The bug causing the chest infections hadn't yet hit Jersey, which, being such a small island has to join in with the UK National Organ Donor register to avoid genetic familiarity. That luck, about which I am so sceptical, was with us this time.

But if we didn't make it to St Mary's Hospital, Portsmouth by 9.30p.m. that same evening, this extremely precious kidney would be wasted.

George and I met in 1981. We married in 1983. He had been married before and when, after two years of going out together and a great deal of impatient frustration, I resorted to asking him to marry me, I'd already thought long and hard about what marriage to George would entail. Twice, he'd tried to propose to me and then chickened out. He'd obviously been doing a lot of deep thinking too! We knew we were in love. We knew we were meant to spend our lives together. We also already suspected there would be no children of our own. Even then there were medical problems which made that virtually impossible. But the medical problems, then, were mine. So the only consideration for me would be whether I could live with him whilst being a distant stepmother to his young son and daughter.

Why do I say "distant"? I certainly don't mean emotionally because I loved and accepted his children from the moment I first met them. No; I mean physical distance. Distance has always been an over-riding problem for our family because George and I live so far away from those we love the most. It causes its own unique set of problems. We met working in Jersey and we live there to this day. Jersey is a self-governing British Island situated about thirteen miles from the coast of France. There's a whacking great stretch of water between Jersey and England and it's called the English Channel.

I am originally from Worcestershire, where my mother still lives. George was brought up in Berkshire. At twenty one he qualified as a Chartered Accountant, married shortly afterwards and had his children, Richard and Kirstie, by his first wife. He came to work in Jersey after his marriage broke down. Five years later, we met. He could earn more money in Jersey, living with his mother who had retired there, than he ever could in England. It meant he would see his children less, but be able to support them more. Richard and Kirstie were always his prime consideration. He trusted his first wife to bring the children up well. It was his job to provide the money so she could do it.

It was to prove a two sided, hard headed, practical solution that both hurt him emotionally and proved a life saver for him because he ended up in Jersey.

Jersey provides only acute and emergency free health care. For everything else, including routine visits to the GP, we are expected to pay. Most people try to take out Private Health Insurance. Without it, we, personally, probably would not have got him to see the experts he needed to see so fast. It gave us both choice and speed and speed has proved essential for treating the illnesses George has.

Just after we met in 1981 George underwent a routine Insurance Medical for work. Hypertension was found and he was advised to give up smoking. In mid-1982 renal impairment was suspected. He was thirty five years old. The Consultant Nephrologist decided to adopt a "wait and see" strategy as he had sufficient kidney function to live a healthy life. We were told to go away and thoroughly enjoy our married life, which we did, with gusto.

George was building his own accountancy practice. I worked in Human Resources, mainly training. Jersey was a booming, exciting place to live and we loved living there. Through living in Jersey, I was able to start building my writing career, first as a hobby, then with a series of random twists and turns which eventually brought success. My love of film and writing for the screen was to be born in those sun-filled days when we were newly married. Jersey was a place where many well-known entertainers came to work the season. The long running BBC television series, Bergerac, was being filmed. Actors, producers, directors, lived alongside us and we made friends with them.

In December 1985, George went on a business trip to Worksop. He came back with first-hand stories of the Miner's Strike, which was then nothing more than news items on the TV to us. He also came back with some impaired vision. "I think I'll go have my eyes tested. I've been doing too much close work."

Christmas always seems to be a time of crisis for us! Christmas 1985 my Mum and Dad were over visiting us for a month. On the day of George's appointment with the optician, Mum and I were in town Christmas shopping. We'd arranged to meet George to get a lift home afterwards. Dad was left at home decorating the Christmas tree. By tea-time, and after being tracked down in town by friends who frantically rang from one shop to another until we were found, Mum and I were in the private wing of the General Hospital to where George had been admitted after being sent from Optician to Eye Consultant to Cardiac Consultant in rapid succession.

"The hypertension is accelerating far too fast. He might not make the next twenty four hours," the Cardiac Consultant, Bill Ginks, told me.

"Could it be Lupus? His sister in Canada's got Lupus," I asked in a panic and was told in no uncertain terms that it was the Consultant's job to do the diagnosis. It is to Bill Ginks's credit that he quietly listened to me that day and started treating George accordingly, although it took another eighteen months for Systemic Lupus Erythematosus to be finally confirmed.

When Mum and I went in to see George in his room, we couldn't believe what we found. He didn't look ill. He looked his normal self. He'd been told to remain in bed, but as soon as I went in, he shot out. "Lie down! You're supposed to lie flat." I hissed.

"Sort this out," he replied, much embarrassed and struggling to retain his modesty. He was wearing nothing but a miniscule hospital gown which he'd put on back to front. He couldn't quite cover his manhood. "I can't let a nurse see me like this."

George is the strong but shy type, a real gentleman who would never wish to offend anyone. He didn't want anyone to see his nakedness unnecessarily. He had used some common sense. He'd tried to keep the gaping flap of the gown designed be worn at the back closed by tying his very conservative business tie around his waist, but it wasn't doing a very good job. Nor did his black knee length socks enhance the overall look. A quick swizz around of the gown by his nervous wife quickly sorted him out.

SLE causes an overactive immune system. It's far less common in men than women. In those days, the doctors were quoting something like ten to one, and we were told that it could present itself in many ways. It often showed itself as arthritis, but if it attacked a major organ and killed it, then it could go into remission.

SLE changed our lives. We had seen how severely, Mag, George's sister who lived in Vancouver, suffered from it. The doctors kept telling us it was just bad luck two siblings on two continents had it as they did not think it was hereditary or familial. Possibly that's the day I started distrusting luck in relation to anything medical. Whatever the chances of getting it were, we knew George didn't want to have it.

It also changed our thinking and our hopes. We started making plans for our future. If George's life expectancy had just gone way down, we had two children to think about and if he was to live, but need a great deal of care, we wanted to be independent, to make our own choices about where and how he was treated. For that, we would need a lot of money.

We started saving money – damned hard! And, unlike many of our contemporaries, from that day forward we made sure we never bought anything we couldn't afford.

We never lost our sense of perspective. What was left over went either on the children, or us. So, as long as all the bills were paid and the family well looked after, George and I decided we were going to enjoy every minute of our marriage for as long as we possibly could. We were going to do all those things we dreamed about. We just agreed we would save up to do them.

But there was one, much more important, thing we learned at that bleak time.

We learned you have to live your life to the fullest, otherwise you make yourself miserable. You have to not think too hard about what can go wrong; because you can be as sure as hell that what you worry about never happens. It's the other stuff that creeps up and makes life really hard for you.

That's what happened with us with the cancer. We honestly, never saw it coming.

Nor did either of us even guess that George was already living with cancer. We'd been lulled into a sense of false security. George seemed so well. But the cancer was so damned quiet and horribly sneaky. It seeks out weakness.

When George had his transplant he was put on anti-rejection drugs, particularly one called Ciclosporin, and all drugs have side effects.

We listened to what the doctors warned us. They told him without some kind of intervention, either the transplant or dialysis; he could have as little as two weeks to live.

The transplant was a life giving gift. Not only did it keep him alive, it gave him the freedom to live his life as he wished.

It was a no-brainer to accept it.

But there's a price to pay. Anti-rejection drugs raise the risk of cancer – and they have to be taken to keep the transplant kidney alive.

You have to be prepared to accept the risk.

The trouble is, over time, the odds became too long for him. The kidney proved to be a good one. It has exceeded all expectations of how long it would last. The average length of life for a transplant when George first received it was about seven years. This one is still going strong sixteen years on. It's remained healthy and appeared to be keeping him healthy. But the longer he had the transplant kidney the more Ciclosporin he had to take. His own kidneys, killed by SLE, as is normal practice, had not been removed. That's where the cancer started growing; in one of his own dead kidneys.

George has always said that his illnesses are his alone. He sees it as his sole responsibility to make any choices regarding how they are treated. He takes advice, listens to the recommendations from his medics and then puts what they suggest into practice.

He's always chosen to go down the conventional medical route. His illnesses have been complex and require a large amount of knowledge to tackle them. It hasn't stopped us looking at alternative medicine. We've just never found anything that would be of use, so we've learned to put our trust in conventional medicine.

Of course there have been times when he has felt thoroughly miserable that he has had to endure so much. All our family have felt with him, but, luckily, those times haven't lasted long. There's always something else going on to distract him.

Bonnie, our family dog, has always been more George's dog than mine and has proved a constant source of quiet but constant comfort to him. Dog and master have that uncanny knack of apparently knowing what each other is thinking. In the mornings, George likes to read the newspaper sitting alongside the window which looks out onto the front garden. Bonnie has a way of just going and sitting alongside him, leaning against his leg and sneaking her nose up under the edge of the newspaper. Inevitably, he puts it down to pat her. I often walk past them on my way into the kitchen and smile at the two of them just sitting, staring out, quite content, seemingly watching the sparrows play in the borders. Sometimes, I wonder if they're actually watching anything at all, they're simply just sitting there companionably.

In Worcestershire we have an old saying:

"Sometimes I just sits and thinks, and sometimes I just sits."

It sums up the pair of them perfectly.

The trouble is; no amount of comfort makes the illness go away. We've found you have to deal actively with cancer to have any chance of leading a happy life. You can't turn your back on it. You have to accept you have got it and get on with it.

At times, it's been hard for our family, but we've all, along with George, learned to accept it. And once you accept cancer, it gets heaps easier to live with. You have to always remember it can happen to anyone. Which is where I think that original question at the top of this chapter needs to be re-evaluated.

The question should not be "Why Him? Why Us?"

You have to think: "Why Not Him? Why Not Us?"

And then you start accepting it.

It's no use ignoring cancer and it's no use thinking it is going to kill you, because, believe me; you never truly know what's going to happen next. George's cancer is incurable but look at how long we've been living with it.

There are still many other things which could happen.. And that – against all the odds – can be incredibly exciting.

CHAPTER TWO

Three Out Of Four People In The UK Get Cancer

Really? Is that absolutely true?

This is one of those catch-all statements that gets blithely bandied around. I suspect it is close to the truth, but who, honestly, is ever going to know the precise number? At any one given time there are people who have been diagnosed and are in treatment, people in remission, people in recovery and people walking around blissfully unaware that this cell malfunction is active within them.

All you can be absolutely sure of is that each patient is completely individual, each patient needs their own diagnosis, all patients will deal with it in their own way and it is very unwise to compare one individual with another.

George and I have learned to be very wary of both the success and horror stories people love to tell with morbid glee.

We've also learned – and proved - never to give up hope because there is always one, often overlooked, element in cancer treatment that can never be measured – the body's ability to heal itself.

George comes from a medical family. Both his parents were doctors, his second sister was a nurse and his older brother was a professor of – you wouldn't believe it! – cancer medicine. Only he and his eldest sister, Elizabeth, broke away from the medical life. George as an Accountant. Liza was a teacher.

Brother Ed, or more correctly, Professor Edward Newlands, late of Charing Cross Hospital, Imperial College and Cancer Research Campaign (Now Cancer UK), who pioneered the development and use of Temozolomide, a chemotherapy treatment for brain tumours, and George were very close. Up until his death in 2006, Ed was always our first port of call to discuss medical problems. Very early on in our marriage, I vividly remember one evening sitting enjoying an excellent meal cooked by my sister-in-law, Liz, in their London home. Ed, slightly red in the face and becoming more voluble with every glass of a very good wine, said "more people live with cancer than die of it."

"What do you mean?"

"We all carry cancer cells. If we could only find out what activates some and not others, then we might have a good chance of finding a cure for cancer."

How that first statement from decades ago stuck with me.

More people live with cancer than die of it.

The more I thought about it, the more I came to understand what Ed was saying. The diagnosis of cancer is not a death sentence. It's a confirmation that there is a health problem. It's a diagnosis which should be acted upon with speed and it is extremely serious; but it isn't necessarily going to be the thing that kills you.

We all know people who enjoy life to the fullest after being treated for cancer. Personally, I have three friends who have now lived over twenty years since they had breasts removed. Each of them says "thank goodness for regular check-ups."

That's the other thing with living with cancer. The threat of its return never goes away.

George and I have talked long and hard in the ten years since he had one of his native kidneys removed in July 2003 with a malignant tumour inside it. The kidney was already unable to function. SLE had seen to that. The tumour grew within an already dead organ. When they took it out, it appeared to be wholly contained within the kidney wall and there was no sign of further spread into the surrounding tissue. Renal Cancer is an odd cancer. It spreads much the same as a dandelion clock releasing its seeds into the wind. It spreads randomly, but for five years we lived in happy bliss not taking much notice of the worry and allowing ourselves to believe that the threat seemed to have gone away.

It hadn't.

Too many other things were occupying our minds. George retired from his business and we took a, fantastic, eight week trip around the world. We hadn't enjoyed ourselves so much for years and we've always been pretty good at enjoying ourselves. Bonnie wasn't yet part of our lives then. We had had another dog, Quincey, who had died at the age of seventeen around six months before and we decided then was the right time to travel for such an extended period.

We wanted another dog, so we planned to look for one on our return. We couldn't believe our luck when we asked at the Vets if they knew of any litters about to be born. "My golden lab is having one in five weeks' time. The father's my boss's Collie. You can have first pick," Donna, the Receptionist and Veterinary Nurse, told us. Quincey had been an all-black, lab/collie cross. We couldn't believe it when this litter, too, all came out black with some patches of white. Bonnie is sturdier in build than Quincey was, but she ended up with a similar, gentle temperament.

I've always thought that that kind, generous personality of hers is a gift that was sent to us in our greatest time of need.

There was so much else going on in that interim period between George having his kidney removed with cancer and the first sign of spread of the cancer in our family too. My dear Dad died at the age of 78 and within a month my Mum, who had been married to him since the age of 19 for nearly fifty two years, met and fell in love with Jim, with whom she still lives. When she was deciding whether they should move in together, she said "I've loved your Dad for all that time and I'll never stop loving him. But if I've loved once, then I can love again." I have never doubted her confidence. Mum and Jim are wonderful together.

At the same time, Kirstie, who we call Koo, met and fell in love with Steve. For many months, usually on a Sunday, I would have first a phone call from my mother telling me how amazing her new man was, quickly followed by a second phone call from my step-daughter saying practically the same thing. Believe me; love knows no age barriers! I'd come off the phone and say to George "we're the meat in the sandwich. Thank God, we're still in love, otherwise I'd be green with envy." In 2007, Koo and Steve gave us our first, wonderful, grandchild, Samuel William.

Then, against all our expectations, Richard, who was enjoying his life in London working as a Film Editor so much he never looked as though he would settle down, fell in love at first sight with Shauna. Three weeks after their first meeting, before we even knew there was a "Shauna" in his life, he nearly gave his father a coronary when, on a Tuesday evening so miserable we'd taken ourselves off to the pub for tea, he left a message sounding terribly anxious and saying he was in Paris, could we please ring him back urgently. When George's hands finally stopped shaking enough for him to dial the number Richard gave, Richard came on the line to say they'd just got engaged. In fact, as far as they were concerned they'd just got married and from that day forward he always referred to Shauna as his wife. On 11.1.11 they gave us beautiful, twin granddaughters, Sophia and Isabella.

Love was everywhere in our family. We didn't have time for illness and we certainly didn't have time to think much about it either.

That was, until that awful day in December 2008, when, during a routine CT on the transplant kidney and what remained of his own native, kidney, the radiographer decided to look a little higher up George's torso. A massive tumour was found sited in the pleural cavity of George's right lung. It was rapidly eating into two ribs and vertebrae. Looking back, he had had symptoms, but they had been dismissed as a strained muscle in his back after he'd been painting the house. How naïve were we!

We had slightly longer to prepare this time, but within four hours we were on a plane to Southampton again. George would have radiotherapy in Southampton General Hospital. This time, unlike the transplant, we seemed to be coping with the awful news rather well. George was admitted onto the ward pending more x-rays. I went off to check into Jurys Inn, the hotel used by Channel Island and Isle of Wight patients who are undergoing radiotherapy.

Five fractions of radiotherapy to the bones were administered and six days later we were back home on the plane in time for Christmas and for George to recover.

I'd already been keeping a diary for a couple of years – not an ordinary "I did this and that and the other today" diary, but a writing diary, my day to day random reminders of where ideas came from, who I've been speaking to, the left-overs which will never get used in my professional work but which have helped to stimulate and inform me.

I regularly read my diaries back because they are a reminder of the type of things which, to me, are memorable, but which have no importance to any particular time, or place, or anyone else.

I enjoy this kind of a journal much more than a diary aimed at forming an historical record. Of course, there are days when I ramble on about the state of the world. To my shame, I moan about the family more than I ever sing their praises. Some days I have nothing to say, but those days really are few and far between. After all, I am a writer and words are the tools of my trade. Primarily I write for the screen. My world is the world of scripts. Every now and again I write script reports, or treatments, but even they have a certain form. Mostly I write scripts in that strict structure used universally for both television and film, so writing in my writing diary feels very different.

I've found a note in one which illustrates more clearly what type of thing I enter. It says:

'This weird looking, giraffe necked, girl at the Wayside had the most beautiful, but tiny, tiny feet, a larger version of a baby's. I think I might give Laura such feet.'

Hardly an entry worthy of Samuel Pepys, but it instantly brings back an image to me and screenwriters do tell their stories in a series of images.

Everyone says "if you want to be a writer, you should write every day." Well, some days you have absolutely nothing worthwhile to say. Those are the days you justify your own existence by writing a few lines in your writing diary!

When the cancer was discovered, I checked back through my diary to see if we had had any warning of it. We had. But we'd missed it. Towards the end of Autumn 2011, I eventually found a tiny entry that reminded me George had had a patch of feeling pretty unwell with backache. On Sunday 13th November, I must have even been starting to get worried, because I wrote:

'And then, today, the pain has eased off and he's cheered up again. He's so stalwart, so accepting. I have to follow his lead and enjoy my day when he enjoys his. So little is discussed nowadays about what makes a good marriage good. All you hear is the bad. But I love being married. You hear women berating men constantly, but I don't want to be like them. I watched my Mum and Dad argue practically every day of my young life. Their marriage seemed to thrive on it, but she stuck by Dad to the bitter end, through illness so devastating, leg amputation, five heart attacks, diabetes, dreadful, dreadful brucellosis. I wanted the love they shared, but I never wanted any of the fighting. We hardly ever argue. I always wanted the quiet respect, support and companionship I've enjoyed with George. We still have great fun together and always put each other first. But the most important thing we retain and maintain is common respect. We say please and thank you to one another. We ask each other's opinion and then respect it. I hear such dreadful ill-mannered behaviour between couples and wonder why they _never_ seem to expect things to go wrong. If only there could be a shift back to the courtesy and romance we heard about tonight on The Antiques Roadshow where love was honoured and upheld through the most dire of circumstances. It was a marvellously moving programme for Remembrance Sunday and I am glad I watched it.'

End of November 2011 and we were travelling in England meeting up with the family; down to London with Richard and Shauna celebrating my sister-in-law, Liz's, 70th birthday, and visiting Mum and Jim for an early seasonal celebration as they had decided not to travel over to us for Christmas this year.

Little did I suspect then quite how much was shortly about to go wrong for all my family – and even my friends.

On Wednesday 30th November, I wrote:

'At Mum's now after what turned out to be an easier journey than I expected. George drove very well, although he does need a navigator as he hesitates more than he used to. Both Mum and Jim have aged since even August and I don't like some of the signs Mum's showing for advanced diabetes. She had a bad fall when they were in Cumbria last week and I think Jim and I are going to have to sit on her to get her to go to see the chiropractor. My stress levels are going to be sorely tested this trip, I suspect. Still, let's just do what we can and take it from there. Bad news from Bonzo who's just found out she has early stage womb cancer.'

Bonzo, Lynne, my longstanding friend of over 30 years, now lives in Grimsby. I would have liked to go to visit her as, over ten months, she first underwent an operation followed by chemotherapy but I never once managed to get there. We still haven't been able to see each other since that day. Within a matter of days things rapidly needed prioritising by me and my ability to travel at will would go out of the window. Bonzo wanted to come to visit us in Jersey but she was advised not to travel by plane for risk of infection. The patch of water between England and Jersey became a barrier and the telephone became essential for me to keep in touch.

I took Mum to the Chiropractor three times whilst we were visiting her. She quickly regained mobility, but by the third session it was obvious something else was wrong. Mum was advised to see her own GP as she was describing pain the Chiropractor couldn't attribute to anything to do with her skeleton.

I visited her GP with her the last day we were staying with them. Mum had got it into her head she wanted to introduce me to her new GP. "If they tell me anything big," she said, "I'll need you to explain it in simple terms to me." Whilst meeting her new doctor, both of us were more than slightly taken aback to find out that now she was living with Jim though not married to him, I, her only child, was no longer regarded as her next of kin. That meant no one would be able to speak to me about her ailments without her express permission. A simple letter to her surgery was all that was needed for them to do it and that, very shortly, proved to be invaluable.

She's also had to give special permission again whenever she's been in hospital. Patient confidentiality is confusing in the way it is protected. It can cause real problems and George and I, only recently, found out that even when you are married, some medical staff will refuse to speak to the spouse without the patient's prior approval; something that proved a real nightmare for us when George was in a state of real confusion.

The GP said she would refer Mum back to the Diabetes Centre first as the pain she was experiencing in her back could be a result of her diabetes. I came back on the plane thinking "Dear God, please don't let this be her kidneys." I thought she was going into renal failure. Cancer was the last thing I expected.

Reading back over my diary, it's noticeable how much more personal the entries became from there on in. It was as though I had started to sense that cancer was about to walk back into our lives and leave lead-heavy footmarks we could never erase.

By Friday 2nd December, I was writing:

I've been thinking about prayer; guiltily rather, because I am a "foul weather pray-er". When things go well I forget to pray, but when things go against my wishes, I dig in deep and ask for help. Is that selfish? Should I always pray thanks for the good things? If so, I must give a huge thank you in my next prayers then for the two hours with Gwyn (Gwyn Garfield-Bennett, my writing buddy) *who has script edited Living with Cherry for me and then another two hours putting her thoughts into the script. I have loved those hours of distraction whilst working at it, thank you.'*

As December wore on, writing malaise set in. I was finding it harder to settle down and complete work even though I had some tight deadlines looming. Monday 12th December was completely indicative of how disaster loomed on the fast approaching black horizon. Bonnie, our dog, was also unwell:

'The wind is blowing itself into a gale. David Cameron and Nick Clegg are at odds over Europe. G & I have had gypy tummies and then Bonnie Dog is sick twice too. I am worried sick about Mum's health. Spoke to both Koo, then Rich and all seems stablish (sic) with them. I think I'm going on mental strike for a while!'

I quite like that word I'd invented - "stablish". Even now I can't think of a better one to express what I was feeling then.

Things got easier over the Christmas holidays. I cooked a fantastic lunch (even if I say so myself) to share with friends and then came this simple entry for New Year's Eve:

'Excellent New Year's Eve at Gio's with Mel and Karen – here's to 2012. May she be brilliant.'

How wrong I would turn out to be!

CHAPTER THREE

2012 – One Hell Of A Year For Olympians

How I hate all those round-ups they do at the end of the year when they make out how fantastic a year it's been! Grudgingly, I concede each year must be magical sometime for someone, somewhere, but 2012 definitely wasn't for me. The fact that 2012 was the year of the London Olympics, which turned out to be both a triumph of organisation and a triumph for the British Olympic team who won more medals than ever before, rather overshadows how dreadful a year it would turn out to be for my family.

I started the New Year with a champagne hangover, bucket-loads of bonhomie and a rigid belief that no matter what happens you have to carry on. Do I think of myself then as being as much a superwoman as those Olympians are? Of course not! I was just trying to carry on as normal.

Sunday 1st January 2012.

'I've always thought of New Year as a non-event but this year, oddly, I have started to think of it as a complete new start. I've written my writing goals and hope to do as well as 2011 – all achieved, bar one. This "new start" philosophy has been compounded by a quote from a strange NZ film, Dean Spurney, we watched this afternoon:-

"The first time something unusual or unexpected happens, it's happenstance. If it happens twice, it's co-incidence. If it happens three times or more, then it's incidence."

This "new start" is becoming incidence in my mind, so I set up (well, I think I have) a new web site for Jan Caston, Writer this morning to make it incidence! I've always resisted "advertising myself" before.'

When January 6th came, we still had little indication what was about to hit us. Mum was still undergoing loads of "opsies" – you know, those tests where cameras invade as many orifices as they can to see what's going on inside. She'd started at the Diabetes Centre, been rapidly referred to what they delightfully called "the stomach man" and the appointments for "opsies" were coming in thick and fast. She accepted every offer of a cancellation which came her way over the festive season. We all knew something was wrong. We just didn't know what. We had to wait and I seemed to do it in a state of blinkered denial. I was up to my neck in work and that was all I allowed myself to think about – well, apart from one extremely important thing.

Friday 6th January

'15 years today since George had his kidney transplant. God bless the family who said yes to donation, to John Wise, the surgeon who did such a good operation, to the many people who have looked after him since. It changed our lives.

I didn't sleep well again last night, so I switched on the computer and wrote to try to meet those deadlines. As a consequence, I've had a day being completely vague and impatient. The wind has died down, so I decided to just do what I could do and because George needed to work on our finances, I haven't been able to get into the office to write at all during the day anyway. Sometimes I feel bereft when I don't write, even a little, but the amount I churned out during my wind howling, sleepless night last night feels as though that counts towards my perseverance – because that's what it feels at the moment writing The Carrols (Don't Do Christmas) – an act of perseverance, certainly not yet pleasure.

By Sunday 8th January, I'd cracked on and broken the back of "The Carrols" but my spirits were in my boots.

Sunday 8th January:

'The weather's settled and so has my agitation. G and I finally managed to make love this morning and the floodgates I've had so firmly sealed until he got stronger were opened so much that I started dreaming of our normal, full relationship again, only to be brought crashing back to earth because the activity has put G's back out again! We're trying so hard to live a normal life, but illness just won't let us. Our love grows as the days slip towards inevitability and we try to make the most of them, sometimes even managing to forget the intense burdens we carry.'

I realise now that this is probably the first time I acknowledge that cancer can kill. Yet, even feeling so low, my writing still pulls me forward. I finished that entry with:

'I read an excellent interview with George Clooney and suddenly an idea for an grown up romance was suddenly there, all based around the "incidence" that my birthday's May 5th, his is May 6th and my first love's was May 7th. I've started to develop it. I think it could be a beautiful story.'

Wednesday 11th January:

'Sophia and Isabella are one today! I can't wait until we see them next week. I hope they've all had a good day. The girls were sicky again yesterday and we haven't heard a word today, so? And, I've learned a valuable lesson, today. The awkwardly shaped temp filling Kiran my dentist did on my tooth fell out 2 hours later as she feared it might. I broke a plate and then G broke Dad's mug. I checked outstanding screenwriting competitions and approaches -
nothing! I booked a trip to Poole for a screenwriting course with Danny Stack in February and forgot it's about an hour from Soton Airport to Poole so I'll arrive late. We went to see The Iron Lady (loved the film). What is happening today? Well, what is happening is I've learned I need to keep pushing. It's no good writing and then doing nothing about it.'

On that day, I really believed all you had to do was keep chugging along. I changed my tune abruptly the next day.

Thursday 12th January

'And today it no longer has any importance at all!

My Mum has bowel cancer.

All my plans I was making must now come to nothing.

Mum has a mountain to come down from.

I have another mountain to climb.

So little is important now, apart from me helping her to deal with what needs to be dealt with.

It may not be the end, but it is part of it.

Once again, my own dreams have to go on hold, but what are dreams compared to the richness of reality? I love my Mum.'

My Mum was dreadfully weepy on that Thursday. She was eighty years old and for the first time, probably ever, she sounded it. George and I lay in bed that night, and he held me as tight as he could as I shed more than a few tears. I suspect his eyes were wet too. We'd underestimated her resilience, though. After I rang her the next day, I wrote:

Friday 13th January.

'We can make no plans until the hospital sets its dates, so the wait continues. Mum is upbeat today. She's set so much in motion, from her hair, her feet, a new will, telling everyone. She's trying to protect me – still! – what else does a good Mum do? My pendulum swings rapidly and to extremes, one swing into intense practicality, then back into deeper anxiety, but overall is a sense of acceptance. What will be, will be and I seem to have very little control over it.'

I was coming to understand the strength of acceptance. None of us is an emotional Olympian. We all have battles to fight. Some of them will be won. Some will be lost. I was learning all over again that only when you accept a situation as terrifying as cancer and look it straight in the face, can you get on and deal with it on a daily basis.

CHAPTER FOUR

Ajay and A.J. – Always Two Of Everything!

My Dad had his first heart attack in 1980, three months after I moved to Jersey to work. It was massive and should, by rights, have killed him. Ninety per cent of his heart was damaged. As she sat beside him in Intensive Care, my Mum was asked if she would like anyone to be contacted for her.

"We've only got one daughter and she lives in Jersey. Are you allowed to ring her in Jersey?" she asked.

When they said they could, she said "I'll have to get her to come home" and what the nurse replied that day set a precedent we would use whenever critical illness hit our family.

"Not just yet. Your husband will only think he's dying. As soon as he wakes up, we'll get her to speak to him on the phone instead."

This was in the days when a pay telephone on a trolley had to be wheeled alongside the patient playing out a long extension wire as it went.

On Sunday and Wednesday, at nine o'clock in the evening precisely, for five weeks, the trolley would be wheeled over to Dad's bedside and I would ring up to speak to him. I was told to keep the calls short and to stay upbeat. Afterwards I would ring my Mum to tell her how I found him. Needless to say, I constantly badgered her to allow me to go home to see him.

"Not just yet," she'd say firmly as if it was a talisman she was hanging on to tightly. "Remember the nurse said he'll only think he's dying." He was terribly ill, had to have two more operations, but was slowly recovering.

Staying away then was the hardest thing I have ever been asked to do and I was on the first plane I could get when I knew he was going to be discharged. I couldn't have been more surprised when he told me he'd guessed exactly why I hadn't gone home to see him. I thought I'd fooled him.

"Didn't you want to see me?" I fretted. This was my Dad and every instinct had been for me to get back to see him any way I could, so I was pretty upset, and actually a bit guilty, at agreeing to stay away.

"What could you have done sitting by my bedside, ducks?" he said. He always called Mum and me "ducks". "There was hardly any room in Intensive Care. They even had to keep asking your Mum to go out if they needed to do anything for me. And, anyway, your Mum was right. It would have frightened me if you'd rushed home. I would have thought you thought I was dying and I wasn't prepared to do that yet. No, your Mum needs you more now I am at home, helping to look after me, than she did when I was in the hospital."

One of the things I think we forget nowadays is that patients in hospital need their rest and that too many visitors can put too great a demand on them. I've sat beside George's bedside more hours than I care to remember and often I've sat there in silence. He hasn't always wanted to talk but he has wanted my presence. Even now, I always ask him to tell me when he wants me to leave.

I've seen visitors around patient's beds treating it as though it is a party. I've seen children allowed to run around wards with little regard for other patients. If a patient is dying, then it's a different thing entirely, you must be there to say your goodbyes, but if they're not dying, I've often thought that quick visits to hospital are the best idea and to leave longer visits for when the patient comes home. After all, who are you really doing it for – the patient or yourself?

So, I still think, that nurse that day thirty three years ago gave us invaluable advice.

Sadly, we've had too many times to put that advice to good use. George has been in six hospitals in England for specialist care. Often, whilst George was in one hospital, my Dad was in another.

My Mum and I have, with great resignation, come to accept it as a given – if there's one member in the family ill, then there's sure as hell going to be another. In 2012, it's been both my husband and my Mum, and even the dog got cancer that year too; but more on that later.

It wasn't confined to just my Dad and George. On 27th July 2003, I had two phone calls within one hour of each other, telling me first George and then my godfather and Uncle, Bert, both had cancer. George was rushed to Guy's Hospital, London. Uncle Bert was taken into Worcester Royal Infirmary. I couldn't leave George to go up to Worcester to see Uncle Bert. Six days later Uncle Bert was dead. On the day of his funeral, which I dearly wanted to attend to pay my last respects, I had no choice than to accompany a very sick and sore

George back on a plane to Jersey. Fog was forecast and he was desperate to get home.

It proved, only too clearly to me, that when it comes to being a relative of someone with cancer, you can only do as much to help them as you are able to do. Never feel guilty if you can't be with them. Circumstances sometimes prevent you from being in the place you want to be at the time you need to be.

Not all co-incidences are unpleasant. For many years George has been a patient in the care of Consultant Nephrologist, Dr Ajay Kumar. Ajay's wife, Dr Kiran Kumar, is our dentist. George and I are supporters of the local Kidney Patients charity, so Ajay and Kiran, who also support them, have become great friends over the years. Sometimes, when we have dinner with them, I do wonder if they are looking us up and down to see if they can see anything else wrong, but I remember, as George's brother Ed would have told us, they are perfectly capable "of leaving the doctoring at work" when they are out socially.

But when George was referred by Ajay to the Consultant Oncologist, Dr Amanda Jones, at Jersey General Hospital in December 2008, it took a while for it to sink in that she was also referred to by her team as A.J.

Because both physicians treated George at the same time, from there on in we found ourselves frequently getting confused and having to say things like "no, your A.J., not Renal Ajay said...".

As the days in January 2012 slipped by and dates for Mum's operation to remove the bowel cancer were firmed up, George was still coping without the targeted chemotherapy which had been started in January 2008 when renal cancer had been found sited in the pleural cavity. Renal cell carcinoma, at present, cannot be eradicated, but it can be controlled. One of the latest drugs available, Sunitinib (trade name Sutent) is usually taken one tablet a day for four weeks, followed by two weeks off, for the remainder of a patient's life.

In January 2008, Sunitinib had been licensed for use in England and our sister Island, Guernsey, but it hadn't yet been added to the prescription list in Jersey although it was agreed by NICE.

It then cost £2,000 per month and Amanda Jones asked if we had any way to fund it. George still had Private Medical Insurance, but his policy had severe exemptions imposed on it. To give Aviva their due, right from the first phone call they were incredibly understanding and the service they have given us since has been extremely supportive. Within two days they had agreed to cover the cost of the drug for six cycles with a review at the end, but for those two days whilst they made their decision, George and I were frantically working out our budgets to see if we could fund it ourselves.

Cancer always hits a patient and their family financially. Luckily, I'm self-employed and I work from home, so I am on hand to look after George, to literally become his Carer, although I never call myself that. I refuse to be called anything but his wife.

But whilst George was at his most ill, I got no work done at all and, subsequently, was unable to earn anything. Our financial decisions thirty years earlier were finally paying off. We had enough money to weather the storm and to pay for the drug if needs be. The cushion from worry was a great comfort.

I've often wondered how people in a worse financial situation than ours cope. Mum and Jim have now lived on their pensions for a very long time and they have to be careful with their money. They are independent and loath to ask for help, but when Mum started to be treated for cancer, we realised she would need a cleaner to take some of the burden off Jim.

Jim and I had already wondered how she would handle such a big operation. We wanted to make things as easy as possible for her. She had been through so much with my Dad and she was determined "they'll never get me into that place unless it's absolutely necessary," meaning the hospital.

The first visit with her surgeon put paid to any fears we had that she would be unwilling to undergo the operation.

I got a phone call as soon as she got back from meeting Mr Pandey for the first time.

"What's he like?" I asked.

"Oooh, he's lovely. I think he's from Nepal. Put one of those hats on him and he'd just be a Ghurkha."

Believe me, that comes from my Mum with the highest praise. My Dad worked all his life for the Royal British Legion doing welfare work. He had a very high opinion of the Ghurkhas which Mum shares. Phew – first problem solved. Mum really liked her surgeon.

"Is he from Nepal?" I asked Jim.

"Don't know. But he's already got your Mum wrapped around his little finger," Jim told me. "As soon as he told her she was wonderful for her age and that he hadn't expected her to pass all the tests they do to work out who can have the operation, she'd have done anything he suggested. He's clever. He's worked her out. He's including her, not just treating her. He's told her it's her job to get better once he's done his job, and you know your Mum, now she's got something to do, she'll get on and do it."

A second meeting and she was raving about this Mr Pandey even more. I suspected she'd already fallen a little in love with him. "He's so funny," she told me. "He always calls me Mrs High. He called Jim, Mr High and when we told him we weren't married and Jim was Mr Hobby, he was ever so cheeky. He asked me if Jim was my hobby!"

"What's his first name?"

"S - something. I don't know. I 'spect he's got one of those long names the Ghurkhas have. You know the ones with all those letters in them."

When I checked him out on the hospital website I fell about laughing. His first name is Steve. "Don't you dare tell him you think he's a Ghurkha," I warned. "Not unless you tell him how much you admire them too."

"Oh, he already knows that!" came the off-hand reply.

The money side proved to be far more of a nuisance. In the days prior to her operation, at a meeting to assess all her needs, someone who should have known better blithely told her "you've got too much money coming in. You'll never get any help," and she believed them.

Jim and I had to handle the anger. "How do all them layabouts keep getting hand-outs, when us who really need it can get none? Look at that Arab with the hook. Came here to kill us and now we're paying to look after him."

The anger had to come at some time. Cancer makes you angry.

George and I visited later in January, combining it with a visit to see the twins after their first birthday. That evening I wrote:

Saturday 21ˢᵗ January

'We spent the day with Mum, a Mum who is so worried, a diminished Mum, a Mum who is talking brave but no longer talking like my Mum. All pretence of her being the strong one protecting me is gone. In its place is the need, the need of the aged parent become dependent on her child. I am sick of this pendulum we seem to have got stuck on, this slicer that swings back and fro, wielding damage, severing, changing, never still, always re-arranging. Tomorrow we see our twin babies and I shall hug them for Mum as she has asked me and I shall hurt the more because she should be hugging them herself. G is being solid, reliable, calming. I am trying for both our sakes

to act like a grown up when inside the child in me is crying with fear of the
unknown. I hate bloody cancer.'

Before we'd left Jersey, I'd forced the issue over what help they could get. I persuaded Jim the information Mum had been given seemed all wrong, so I asked him to go to see the MacMillan representatives in the hospital. He explained the situation and was reassured we were indeed right and the first person had been wrong. I filled the ample forms out for them during that visit and within a few weeks Mum had been awarded Carers Allowance which covered the cost of a cleaner and took an enormous amount of pressure off Jim whilst she was undergoing chemotherapy.

I have the hugest respect for the MacMillan cancer support and particularly their cancer nurses. As a family, we've had advice from all the major cancer charities either in the form of booklets, through talks and through representatives, but the MacMillan nurses have been rocks when we have needed them.

As the rest of January dragged on and Mum seemed to be required at the hospital for one test or another every day, the rest of the family were having problems too. In Northampton, the twins were teething and kept getting stomach infections. Isabella ended up in hospital to be rehydrated. Poor Shauna had months of living "in the twilight zone" as she called it, as not only the twins, but Richard and she had repeated gastric flu too.

Meanwhile, Kirstie had other problems. She'd been made redundant early in January with only a week's notice, another victim of the recession. By early February she had another job, but it wasn't starting straight away and she would need to do some retraining at her own expense to take it. George and I sent her the money. She and Steve couldn't find that much all in one go with all their everyday commitments. Again, thank goodness our savings meant we had it to give to them.

So, early in 2012, George, who was off chemotherapy and doing well, was taking a bit of a back seat. In fact, he'd been taken off chemotherapy early in 2009. Why and what happened back then was odd. I still can't quite get my head around what I witnessed. And it all had to do with Bonnie.

Six months after he started Sunitinib, in July 2008, she started sniffing around his left ankle as if there was something really interesting there. "Have you had a shower this week?" I teased him. "Or have you been dropping food down you again?"

"It always hits my big belly first. You know that," George retorted. But it worried both of us that the dog was showing so much interest in always the same area of his leg. It was as if she was trying to tell us something was going on around there.

Nothing appeared for several days. Then, one night as he undressed for bed, he found the very first visible signs of something unusual in the area she kept sniffing. There were two, very tiny, spots which looked nothing worse than red freckles, one just above the ankle and the other higher up inside the calf. More worrying was that they were weeping.

The dog was right to alert us.

Ajay Kumar was concerned it was another site of renal cancer, which can spread anywhere in the body. Biopsies were done but have never proved conclusive. As the wounds were healing, we had one of the hottest spells of the year. The wound nearest the ankle broke down and over time, became ulcerated. By February 2009, Amanda Jones felt George was doing well enough that he could have a "chemo holiday". It still took many months of specialist care – and a healthy dollop of Manuka Honey, for that ulcer to start healing. Subsequent and regular CTs and MRIs persuaded Doctor Jones that George could manage without the chemo.

To all intents and purposes, in January 2012, he was doing well. We were being lulled into a false sense of security. Anyway, we had other major things on our mind. We had my Mum battling bowel cancer. And George was more worried about her than he was about himself.

Waiting for dates to be firmed up for Mum's operation the fears were all for my Mum. Then quite out of the blue, more, totally unexpected, problems hit us.

Monday 30th January

'The tears came this morning. They had to come at some point. So on a cold and miserable morning I worked like a Trojan to get on top of things and exhausted myself, had to complain again about our drains – blocked again!, ate too much comfort food, slept and worried. I hate this bloody waiting.'

Tuesday 31ˢᵗ January

'January has finished on another sour note. Bonnie was bitten by one of the farm's Alsatians this morning and has had to have ten stitches in her flank. She's okay, lucky really, but it meant all morning was taken with sorting her out at the Vet Hospital. Then we saw Amanda Jones in the afternoon about George. Chest x-rays appear to remain stable, so more checks in six weeks and no chemo again, thank God. We finally got Bonnie back, very doped up, from Hospital about 7.30, ate a quick bite then got a phone call from Mum fretting because she's still heard nothing about her dates today and they did say they'd phone her by the end of last week.'

We'd taken Bonnie for a walk on public land, a mixture of fallow fields and cliff path. She loves to run and chase her ball there. The Farmer farms some fields alongside and that morning he was feeding his pigs as we passed. His three Alsatians were with him, but loose. Two of them completely ignored us, as they always had in the past, but the third watched Bonnie running for her ball and for some reason decided to chase her. The trouble was, she didn't go for the ball. She went for Bonnie and brought her down. Bonnie did what all the members of our family do when under attack. She got back on her feet and she ran for her life. We're not stupid. None of us Newlands hang around to fight fights we can't win! Luckily she was far faster than the Alsatian who then casually trotted back to re-join the Farmer.

We had no idea Bonnie was so badly hurt. She carried on chasing her ball until the end of the walk and it was only when we were putting her into the back of the car that we saw this great gaping wound opening up. It was a tear from where a very sharp tooth had gone in, about six inches long, but clean, through the upper layer of her skin which holds her fur. Luckily, it hadn't penetrated any lower section skin or muscle.

We rushed her to the Vet's where she was injected with antibiotics and then taken to the Vet's Hospital for stitches. She came home with a "bucket" on her head to stop her gnawing or licking her stitches and she was very down in the mouth for several days. She even went off her food and that's very unlike Bonnie who has so much Labrador in her.

We showered her with affection and put all our energy into looking after her. George was particularly concerned about his "little girl", but not as much as the Farmer who even offered to have his Alsatian put down. We felt, the Alsatian couldn't really be blamed. It was only doing what it is bred to do; protect its land. The Farmer paid our Vet's fees and has kept the dog close to the farmhouse ever since. It hasn't stopped me being scared of the dog though.

Mum didn't get her dates until Friday 3rd February. The operation was scheduled for 24th February and we were due to depart on a ten day cruise from Southampton on the 23rd. Cancelling that turned out to be a fiasco too. We agonised over what to do. George and I badly needed a holiday. We left it until the very last minute to decide, cancelled and arranged to contact our travel insurance company, only to get an email from the cruise company two hours later to say they had Norovirus on board and if we wished to alter our arrangements, we could. When I rang them and explained what had happened, they refused to re-arrange for us as we had already cancelled. Couldn't they have told us there were already problems when I rang! But, hey, no, they were adamant. Never have I wished I'd waited another two hours to make a phone call more! I certainly don't think I'll be using that particular company ever again!

Life was certainly busy, but George and Mum seemed to be coping well. On Thursday 9th February I even managed to make my trip, on a bitterly frosty, cold, day to Poole to listen to Danny Stack talking about being a Director and how to write for T.V. George was left in charge of a still miserable Bonnie. That day for me, talking about writing, turned out to be the only short day of relief for some time to come.

Bonnie came for her evening treats on Sunday 12th February and I noticed her face seemed misshapen. We took the first appointment of the morning at the Vet the next day in case she was having an allergic reaction to the antibiotics they'd given her following the bite.

Monday 13th February:

'It's been a horrible day for Bonnie. She was rushed into the Vet Hospital again to have a lump cut out from under her eye by Ben Linnell. He's done such a neat job in a very awkward area but all evening she's cried with pain. When we collected her, her eyes were awash with 'tears'. It was heart-breaking. It's not been such a great day for me either. I had a very polite rejection from the contact I made and had set my hopes on this being 'the big one'. All in all, mid-afternoon, I had the shakes through a combination of sadness for Bonnie, worry over Mum and George and resigned exasperation for my own dreams. I have so much I want to do, but this phase of being needed by everyone else and not being able to get on with my own life just will not budge.'

Bonnie had mast cell cancer and we were lucky it had shown up so quickly. It's another cancer which acts completely irrationally. Lindsey Linnell,

Ben's wife, who is also a Vet in the practice, put her on chemotherapy, one tablet given in tinned dog food every four weeks, for eight cycles. Bonnie started her life in this particular Veterinary Practice where she had been conceived and born. So, even before all this started, she was always over-excited about going in there as to her it's like "going home". When she started the chemotherapy she became even worse and she still thinks every time she goes in she will get tinned dog food which we never feed her at home.

Ben and Lindsey also own Bonnie's brother, Jasper, so they were particularly interested in how she would take the treatment. Lindsey and Donna became really clever at finding a way to take the blood they needed to check her progress before each session of chemotherapy. They found that if Donna whispered and blew in her ear, Bonnie would just present a leg for Lindsey to draw the blood drawn off. Dogs are clever. They know what they need to do to get help.

It took eight months of treatment, but at present no other cancer has revealed itself yet. I do, however, religiously check over her well every day when I groom her.

So, whilst we were dealing with all these problems, Mum still hadn't had her operation and that was fast coming up. We did have one delightful bit of respite though. Our grandson, Sam, had started pre-school the previous September, so Koo brought him over to visit for four days of his half-term. From the fuss he made of her, I swear Bonnie thought he'd come over solely because she'd been ill.

CHAPTER FIVE

Keeping Going When Everything Is Falling Apart

Coming up to the date of Mum's operation, it was hard being in Jersey with George unable to travel because he had consultations looming and Bonnie still walking around with a "bucket" on her head to protect her stitches meaning she couldn't possibly go into kennels. I would have dearly loved to have a comfortable chat over a cup of tea with my Mum. The dreaded Norovirus had hit Worcester Royal Hospital and the news was deteriorating daily.

Saturday 18th February

'It's hit me hard today how worried I am over Mum. Worcester Royal now has 12 wards closed to outsiders for Norovirus. She can't have a major op with that level of risk. She said last night "you should have gone on your cruise because I shan't be having the op". What can we do! Bonnie is improving and has stopped crying with the pain. The four frozen peas in a plastic bag Donna (from the Vet's) suggested to press against the stitches and reduce the swelling has helped, thank God.'

It's at stressful times like these; I normally lean heavily on George for support without even thinking. When someone's ill themselves, you start being aware that there are times when you simply cannot rely on them anymore.

Sunday 19th February

'There was a point, undressing for bed tonight, when George and I stopped to listen to something on the news on telly. We sat on the edge of the bed and we were like two peas in a pod. At that point I felt such a sense of togetherness. But it was mixed with a dreadful sense of foreboding that something even worse is about to happen. It's awful that I've become so conditioned by everything that's been going on recently that I always expect something bad after experiencing something so good. I'm not feeling sorry for myself. I'm being accurate. Over the past few months, after any intense happiness, the situation has always rapidly worsened. I can no longer take anything for granted.'

This feeling obviously stayed with me for days because on Tuesday 21st February, I wrote:

'George, with all his problems, is still functioning better than me. He seems able to plan steadily, to forge his way through insufferable inconveniences. He is so strong mentally and I really admire him for that. In fact, I admire him for everything he's achieved. He truly has achieved his full potential.'

The days dragged on. I tried to keep to our normal routine, but the weather was miserable and so was I.

Saturday 25th February – 11.36am.

'I've got a cold. I stayed in bed and finished The Redeemer by Jo Nesbo while George walked Bonnie. I love the Harry Hole character, how his morality, his caring, gives him weakness and balance. He makes me realise my own inadequacies are universal, not individual. I know no man is perfect yet still my own guilt neurones flagellate me into expecting me, personally, to be perfect. I'm currently awash with a mixture of cold germs, neuroses and genuine concerns. It's a foul cocktail and it's contributing to making me woozy and terribly unwell. Why do I allow myself to endure this self-made, pseudo-alcoholism, when I rarely touch a drop of the actual stuff which might, just, cheer me up? Perhaps I should start hitting the bottle!

Two days ago when I moaned like mad that the three "people" I love the most have cancer, George, who lives with it, dealing with it so deftly, so lightly, said, "That proves it right then, does it? That three out of four people will get cancer."

That makes me ashamed and the pain of it is manifesting itself in my hand. My fingers tingle. My thumb hurts holding the pen. My breathing has shallowed. I can feel the air struggling its way into my right lung.

I'm frightened.

And I'm not only scared witless for the only three people I love as they battle this demon called cancer.

I'm frightened I'm going to get it myself.

And seeing what I've seen of the suffering people have to go through to deal with it, I'm terrified that when it's my turn I shall be a coward.

So much for the brave words I'm churning out to reassure those three people I love the most! This is too damned real and it leaves me in a mental state of paralysis.'

Thank God, a good lie in bed and paracetamol helped me to feel much better later in the day! I had obviously started to regain my equilibrium because by 10.06pm (precisely!) I wrote:

'When I read back the heartfelt words I write, often when I'm at my lowest, I realise what a catharsis it is to be able to express them. As the day's gone on, I've felt better. I've come past that bleakness and emerged on fresher ground. I've still got the sorest, reddest nose though! This compliment of cancer is, quite literally, causing an open ended saga. We've all been battered badly, but we're still here, still fighting, still moaning because we have a right to moan, but no right to give up. Life is just too precious.'

You must never give up. Mum was told to ring the hospital to confirm they had a bed at 10am the next morning. When she rang, they still couldn't tell her. We had a whole day waiting. It was purgatory, but by the time I went to bed that night, we had turned an important corner.

Sunday 26th February

'Mum finally got a bed in hospital at 7pm tonight. She's on her own for now in a 2 bed bay and will not be allowed visitors due to Norovirus, so even if I'd been able to get over to be with her, I wouldn't have been allowed to see her. I was able to ring though – thank God, for the phone – and she's amazing. "I've got the nurses to chat to," she says "and my gardening book". The op is scheduled for tomorrow afternoon, so no news until Jim can ring after 6pm. It will be a long day.'

Monday 27th February

'Mum had her op this afternoon and when Jim rang she was still in the Surgical Dependency Unit, so we won't really know much until tomorrow

lunchtime after the rounds. I've been much calmer than I anticipated. Particularly after having such an awful night's sleep. There's not much to say really. It will all become clearer as the week goes on and we get through Bonnie's blood test tomorrow as well.

George is getting on my nerves, a sure sign I'm needing him to be less dependent. When this stressful period is over, I won't feel that way, but for now, I do.'

George always says being the patient is much easier than it is to be the one who can only sit and give support. At least the patient knows what they are expected to do and get on and do it.

My 80 year old Mum, as ever, was amazing, but nowhere near as amazing Mr Pandey. He managed to remove ten inches of her upper bowel and to do a full reconstruction, all by laparoscope. She was in hospital three days for a major operation and discharged on the fourth. I relaxed a little.

Wednesday 29th February

'We needed a break. G took me to see The Best Exotic Marigold Hotel this afternoon. The cinema was three-quarters full and the film was an absolute tonic. If only I could write like that!"

The come back down to earth wasn't so easy for me, particularly when I took a phone call two hours before I got on a plane to go to see Mum. George was well enough for me to leave and I arranged for friends to pop in to check on him and the dog. The last thing I needed when I was in such a rush was to get a call saying our Private Health Insurance was about to lapse as the credit card the broker had submitted had expired a year before. I'd reminded them to change it when we renewed it a month before. They'd obviously forgotten to update it. The last thing I wanted was for our Private Health Insurance to lapse.

Thursday 1st March

'My amazing Mum came out of hospital at 10.30 this morning. 80 years old and she has a major op and she is out within three days – unbelievable.

And there am I! By 10.45 I was having a screaming fit at the computer, my stress levels had reached blowing time. But it was the best thing I could do. I need to let off steam because even today when I could do with everything going smoothly things are going wrong with that damned Insurance again. I thought I sorted it all out last year. Even George agreed that the first two months of this year have been so stressful, he's exhausted. But George has a technique where he can shut himself down and calm down. I need to blow and it's best if I do it at inanimate objects like I did this morning.

At the moment I'm praying for a little light wind. It's very mild and that's causing fog. I just don't want to sit at the airport tomorrow, so perhaps a Force 2-4 would be good. This is the constant problem with an Island on the edge of the Atlantic. But when we drove around Corbiere this morning after taking the dog for a short walk, it looked so romantic with the low rocks shrouded in mist and the lighthouse peeping out above the mist reflecting the bright sun back over a gently flowing sea, my anxiety settled.

I watch the news and for weeks it's all been about civil unrest in Syria with bits about the protests in Cairo and I heartily thank God that I was born in beautiful, rural Worcestershire, then moved to exceptionally pretty Jersey. It'll be 33 years this year. Such a long time but I can't complain I've been short changed with the places I've lived.

When I go to London nowadays I see it only as bricks and mortar, too many people competing for too little, grubby, space. People say they could never live in the countryside, preferring an urban life because it's livelier, more exciting and that there are more opportunities.   That argument defeats me. We don't do so bad here, do we? They prefer never to walk in a straight line on a pavement, to cycle amongst engine fumes, to sleep with never ending light and sirens, sirens, sirens. How can that cause anything but stress? I walked with G and Bonnie this morning and for the whole of the 40 minutes I saw only one man and his dog. I listened to the spring chattering of birds, came home to see daffodils and crocus, scylla and hyacinths, all out below our stunning camellias in their ball gown dressage.

If I have to lose my temper because life has been so difficult, I'd rather do it in surroundings like that. I may be feeling unwell with my sinus, worried about my beloveds having cancer, but I still have comfort. Thank God, I have eyes to see it.'

I talk a lot about God because I believe in God. George doesn't. He believes there is no other life than what we get in this one. I believe when we die we go on to a better place.

George believes we become nothing; though since he watched a programme on the Large Hadron Collider at CERN searching for the Higgs bosun he's latched onto the idea of becoming a quark when he dies and shooting around the universe faster than the speed of light. When I told him quarks are believed to be able to go through any other type of matter without it feeling them, he got quite excited at the prospect of being able, if he became a quark, to shoot through me and the children without us knowing he was there.

Sometimes I wonder what drugs he is actually on!

And I asked him how he thought he had any chance of becoming a super-quick quark when in this life he is so slow and placid. We laugh about it often. Laughter is a central element to our married life.

We got married in the Royal Court of Jersey, which sounds rather regal until you realise it was then a pokey room in which our marriage was legalised in two sentences in a civil ceremony. I wanted to be married in Church, to take my vows, but I wasn't allowed to take them in a full marriage ceremony as George had already been married in Church and had broken his vows with his divorce. Wedding vows were treated as more binding thirty years ago. I felt angry that I was being denied the right to take them when I had done nothing wrong apart from falling in love with a man who had seen such a sad end to his early, first marriage. The best we could hope for was a blessing. I grudgingly agreed to settle for the civil ceremony in Jersey if nothing else to keep down costs.

I've watched the arguments going on in Parliament and the Anglican General Synod about allowing a full marriage ceremony for same sex couples and my heart aches. I understand only too well how people feel when they are told "no, this is the Law" because I had no alternative way back then than to accept it. I understand the depth of rejection, the hurt that the togetherness you feel cannot be sanctified.

I often wonder if perhaps the argument has gone in the wrong direction; that it's all about the legality rather than the long term benefit. I wonder if instead of a one size fits all approach to marriage, which, after all, is in religious terms for the procreation of children, that a new form of "taking vows" could be found for same sex couples to sanctify their civil partnership.

I can vouch for marriage. It's wonderful. It gives your relationship a depth which is extremely rewarding, particularly in times of stress, but, to me, marriage in church gives you no more legal right than a civil ceremony. I think the argument's trying to force a form of acceptance, but who is the acceptance to come from? God? My God would be having a laugh at our expense for us getting "our knickers in a twist" over this one. In France, the Mayor marries you in a civil ceremony and then you go to Church for the marriage to be blessed. That seems to work.

Back then, I was prepared to respect and accept the ruling. So, when the rector of Mum and Dad's local church in Worcestershire offered to bless our marriage, both of us were delighted. Canon D'Oyle first offered to do it in Church, but then he came up with a much more personal solution. My grandfather had only just died and had been buried on December 13th. Canon

D'Oyle suggested that as I was the last person to be born in the house where my family had been born for four hundred years before me, from where my grandfather had made his final journey before he was buried and which my parents would soon be leaving before it was sold out of the family, it would be a nice idea if he blessed our marriage in the house on Boxing Day 1983.

I felt that day that my marriage had indeed been blessed and looking back I've often thought that the solution couldn't have been more perfect for George and me. It was very, very special indeed.

Neither of us had ever met Canon D'Oyle, but we were told that the children at the local infants' school where he took assembly called him "Can of Oil". Dad told me how he had the biggest laugh over it. We liked the sound of the man but we thought that, out of respect, we ought to tell him that neither of us went to Church although we were both confirmed Anglicans and that only one of us still believed in God.

We took a long time writing the letter thanking him for his kind offer. It took us over three hours of deep discussion to decide how to describe George's beliefs. We had no idea that what we wrote as we lay, together, naked, in bed on a Sunday morning would subsequently be quoted in one of his sermons. George really does believe "seeing is believing" so eventually we decided on describing his beliefs as "agnostic with reservations". Over the years, how we've come to regret that turn of phrase!!! We're still being teased about it.

This all makes me sound a bit "holier than thou" which I'm certainly not; but I do have a faith based on the power of prayer. Don't ask me where it's come from. I've just always felt it and I'm truly glad I do.

It's very unfashionable to say that, isn't it?

I don't find God in Church. I find him everywhere and He's with me all the time. My "Church", if you want to call it that, is the space on the edge of the headland above Beauport Bay in Jersey from which you can see four other bays in a horseshoe and where the sky always feels like a never ending canopy drawing you in to safety. That's where I go when I feel I need to. I walk there with Bonnie and as she sniffs around the gorse checking for birds' nests, whilst there, I find peace and understanding.

That's so important when you are the relative of someone dealing with cancer. You have to have a break from the grinding reality of living with cancer. You have to look after your own needs as well as the patient's. For me, retaining a healthy sense of my own spirituality, keeps me sane. For other people, it will be doing other things.

It's all a case of finding what you need to help keep you going and making sure you get it.

CHAPTER SIX

The Absolute Pits: Part One

In Worcestershire, Mum was due to start chemo in April but hadn't yet got her dates. In Jersey, Bonnie was still enjoying her visits to the Vets for her chemo "breakfast" and her bloods were coming back just "on the right side" of normal. The two day wait between when the bloods were taken and the results arriving was always a long one. She was certainly recovering her appetite and stamina and the scar under her eye was slowly "furring over".

In Grimsby, Bonzo, my friend Lynne, was coping well with chemo but had got frustrated with losing clumps of hair so had shaved it all off.   Photos she sent made her look absolutely hilarious. I much preferred to see her "au natural" than with a scarf covering her naked scalp. "So do I", she agreed. I was delighted to see her looking so well.

Then, quite out of the blue, we had a falling out over my impending "big" birthday. Everyone was pressing me to have a party. We had always celebrated in the past and the parties had been great fun.

This time, though, I simply did not feel like celebrating. I couldn't quite get out of the back of my mind that my Dad had died two days before my last "big" birthday and I was dreading the same thing happening again, which, of course, there was always the possibility it could with both Mum and George being unwell.

The family accepted my reticence over having a big party and, luckily, decided not to do anything as a surprise, but they did press me into deciding on doing something where we could all be together. I finally, and very grudgingly, agreed to a simple pub lunch but I told everyone I could only cope with my closest family being invited.

I would have been delighted to see Bonzo. On top of everything else that was going on in my own life, I had been very anxious about her. She couldn't make the lunch. She was working. So she wanted to travel to the Midlands to meet up before it but hadn't realised I wouldn't be back in Worcestershire until four days later than she expected. When I pointed that out, she thought I was putting her off. It was a simple misunderstanding, but I hated the hurt I heard in my friend's voice, particularly as she, too, was facing one of the biggest challenges of her life.

It was a bad time for both of us.

Monday 11th April:

'Mum's still not heard when she can start chemo and this evening I upset Bonzo by telling her I didn't want her to drive all that way to celebrate my birthday when she can't make it for the actual day. Why is my damned birthday a reason for everyone to get so excited! I'm dreading it. I've told everyone I don't want to celebrate it because it brings back bitter memories of losing my Dad and still they don't get the message.

I feel awful about Lynne. The other thing is that Mum's so worked up about this delay to her chemo, I don't think she could take a visitor anyway. And, in all this, poor George – again – is being neglected at a time when he should come first. This is <u>bloody impossible</u>; so many things pulling me in opposite directions. Lynne is so far away it's impossible to know what I can do to help.'

I had to face the fact then that I was being forced to prioritise my time, particularly, the amount of it that I could give to the people I loved.

George, then Mum, had to come first.

I was so agitated that I should be doing "the right thing", I started seeing omens everywhere.

Monday 11th April'

It's 3.30 in the morning and my anxiety won't let me sleep. When I was on the phone to sister-in-law, Liz, yesterday, she had a robin which kept flying into the windows of her conservatory kitchen. We joked it was spring and he was mating, but within minutes a hail storm sprang out of nowhere and was beating against the glass so loudly we had to stop the call. The poor creature must have been desperate for shelter. I know how he feels.'

And what we'd told no one at that point after months of "not too bad" scans for George, who was still off chemotherapy and almost back to his normal self, was that something else had shown up which had to be investigated. George was given an urgent appointment for a P.E.T. Scan in Southampton. Normally, I would have gone with him for the day, but with Bonnie still so unwell, he persuaded me he would be perfectly capable of going alone.

My head told me he was, but my nerves still went through the ceiling, compounded by the fact the scan was booked for Friday 13th April. Now, I'm not particularly superstitious but I was this time over that particular date.

Thursday 12th April

'We're both nervous, trying to be normal, dancing on eggshells in the brave way we have of just trying to get through the day. Oh, how weak I feel, and I'm supposed to be the strong one! But, I still have George and Mum and Bonnie and Lynne and I should be celebrating that – not getting het up about a ridiculous birthday. Mum has rung the hospital and it looks as though she's going to be delayed yet another week "because of Easter". Can't they plan! Didn't they know about Easter? Honestly!

There are no words I can find to be wise or erudite or philosophical or funny. I'm writing because the sheer physical act has become in itself a source of comfort. If I can put one cohesive sentence together then I must be functioning on one level, even if, on the deepest, I'm imploding. Once tomorrow is over and we get G's results, I can start to go forward again.'

Friday 13th April came and went. When I got into bed that evening and reviewed my day, even I was surprised.

Friday 13th April

'G went, it was done and a very tired man came back on an earlier flight. Now we wait for the results, but at least it's done. Mum, too, finally got her dates for chemo and again they said the delay was due to Easter – honestly! In an odd way, I've actually enjoyed my day. It's been a fresh day, so Bonnie and I had a good walk all the way over the headland. She was as mad as a March Hare checking out all the smells. She came back exhausted and slept all afternoon! Typical dog's life, eh! She did have a few quizzical looks at G's chair, then decided he wasn't far away, so settled down. I had to go weekend food shopping. G came home and this evening we accepted a last

minute invite for a curry with Mel and Karen, back from America and bursting
with news about Matthew and Leigh Ann's wedding.'

When I look back, I cannot imagine how we got through all of the cancer
"crap" without our friends.   After our family, they are the people who make our
life worth living and at times we have relied on them to bring the outside world
in to us along with their news. Maintaining friendships becomes really important
when you are restricted by the unremitting invisible chains on your time and
dreams that cancer imposes. But, sometimes, just feeling you are still part of
the world, gives you a little fillip.

Wednesday 18th April

*'Just had a lovely evening with Monty and Sam. George told me to go out
for a few hours. At one point, sitting listening to them talking, I thought how
happy I was to have friends like them. It's been a strange old day – G has just
spotted himself on the local late evening news! We happened to walk past the
end of Bond Street mid-morning just as the Police were putting a man in a
bobble hat into the back of the Police car. Apparently there had been a stabbing
in the Bond. What on earth was going on in a pub at that time in the
morning! G's quite delighted he didn't look too old or fat … oh yeah!!'*

It's amazing how quickly your senses of curiosity, humour and fun
return. It's just a pity reality has to kick in again and spoil the fun.

Once again we were forcibly reminded that what you expect, rarely
happens, so, really what is actually the point of worrying? We had convinced
ourselves George was going back on chemo.

Tuesday 24th April

*'Well, we have George's P.E.T. scan results, but what a fiasco it was to get
them. I cannot believe what little support Amanda Jones got to pull them all
together. The scan has highlighted three areas of concern – the arachnoid cyst
in the brain which was known about and needs nothing doing; a thickening of
the bowel, again mentioned before and which she thinks is probably a polyp so G
now has to have a colonoscopy; and then there are three active areas in the
lung which will need to be discussed further as they don't appear to be renal*

cancer as expected. They could be a different form of lung cancer. She will get the Respiratory Consultant to give a second opinion. If it is something new, Sunitinib will be ineffective so it will be a different treatment again. Dear God, what next?'

Even the weather seemed to be against us.

Sunday 29th April

There's a Force 8 blowing, it's been ghastly all day and when we parked at La Rocque to go to Carol's b'day tea party, the wind blew me – great big me! – off my feet. The weather's imitating what's going on all around. Mum's chemo start has been changed again – getting more confused and fractious by the minute. She's now due to start May 4th (the day before my birthday celebration lunch and my Dad died on May 3rd). Dear God, please don't let history be repeating itself.'

In the end Mum's chemo start was put back even further, to May 14th. It was all starting to take a hell of a toll on me, but in the end, I was spoiled on my birthday trip back to see Mum and even managed to enjoy it.

Thursday May 3rd to Tuesday 8th May

'I was wrong about the exhaustion. I woke Thursday morning, went downstairs feeling woozy and then went back upstairs and suffered real breathlessness and light-headedness. I thought it might have been a panic attack and said nothing to anyone. I was anxious about the journey and keen to get there. It did pass eventually and once I was at Mum's, and had seen how well she is looking, I calmed. Thinking back to what happened, I don't think now that it was a panic attack. It was more physical. I'll make a Doctor's appointment to get my blood pressure checked out tomorrow.

So the big trip came and went and was much better than I had hoped. I was very spoiled. Everyone turned up and we had a good lunch. The worst thing that happened that week was that at one point I felt a bit bored because everyone needed to rest so much. Worcestershire was looking at her absolute best and I would have loved to have got out more to see her again. Says it all, doesn't it? Never satisfied, but it has made me think one thing – when I can; I *shall get out and travel more again. That is my birthday gift to myself – a promise.'*

My wooziness was a problem with medication, which was quickly sorted out. The GP told me it didn't usually present itself like that and I came away wondering if it was actually my brain reminding me I had to remember to look after myself as well as everyone else.

I even started to think the pressure was lifting.

Friday 18th May

'I never thought I'd be recording a quote from Tom Jones, the singer, but here goes "Pressure is only pressure if you can't cope with it." There have been times over the past four years when I've been close to giving up, but every time I've been asked to step up to the line, I do. Tonight I can say how proud I am of myself without my normal, self-effacing, apologising.'

My own work took a turn for the better during this period too. Two commissions I'd submitted were accepted.   I found out I'd been shortlisted for a major writing competition and following on from October 2011 when we had started filming a short film called Togo which a good friend, Sue du Feu, had written and was directing, we were back together to finish filming location and time specific scenes. Sue had asked me to come on board as an Associate Producer, which in reality meant I rushed around finding locations, props, costumes, generally being the factotum/runner and I loved it.

The film is about the final days coming up to the Occupation of Jersey in June 1946. We had got away with the exterior of buildings shoot in October 2011 which had brought spectacularly sunny weather. We were praying the middle of May 2012 would replicate June closely enough so that the trees and foliage looked authentic. It was the only time we could film. The first few days were cold, but the light was good, so we went ahead. The next were forecast to be ghastly, with heavy rain, quite unlike what we wanted. The shoot had to be delayed.

I had arranged a visit to London for George's birthday so it turned out I wasn't able to be there for what became the final days of filming. Luckily, my part in it all, by then, was mostly done. I left them to it.

Just before we left the Island, we had the results from the further investigations following George's P.E.T. Scan. There was a polyp in his bowel which was removed and found to be benign. First "phew" of relief. Then the results came in from the spots on the lung. It was renal cancer, just following an unusual route along scarring from previous radiotherapy. It appeared to be reducing in size so no chemo was necessary. Second "phew"; and as George had had the arachnoid cyst since birth, so there was no need for any further action.

We went off to London with sighs of relief and determined to enjoy ourselves, which we really did. We had dinner at Salieri's in the Strand before going to see the musical, Top Hat. We finished that evening with cocktails in our hotel and in my writing diary I wrote:

Friday 25th May

'I dressed up and felt wonderful – why do people dress down so much when you can feel this good? I felt superb. George ate for England and talked about his relief and _happiness_ at the good results from the hospital. We agreed it's time to start living again. Cocktails after – see - LIVING'

The next day we went to see the Canalettos and Hogarths at Sir John Soane's house and then had a magnificent lunch at Rules behind Covent Garden. As we ate our lunch, we remarked how normal life suddenly seemed.

After London we travelled up to see how Mum was doing in Worcestershire. She was looking really well. We took her and Jim to a favourite restaurant, The Wagon Wheel at Grimley, for Sunday lunch. I could not believe how much food she put away. She'd told me she'd lost weight but I couldn't see it. "She does when she's on the chemo," says Jim, "but she soon puts it back on again when the sicky feeling goes." Mum's always believed good food can cure anything!

After that we travelled down to Thatcham to visit Koo, Steve and Sam. It meant a stay overnight and so as not to make work for them, we stayed in a hotel.

Monday 28th May

'Our time with Koo, Steve and Sam was short but wonderful. Sam remains a delight. He let me bath him after we collected him from school,

giggling all the time. Then, after an early dinner at The Bunk Inn which went on longer than expected, when Koo was starting to worry about ever getting him into bed as it was a school night, we suggested they took us back to the hotel first so Sam could "put us to bed". It worked. Sam led Granddad into the room, made him sit on the bed and proceeded to take his shoes off for him. When he asked Granddad where his pyjamas were, Koo and I had to dive into the bathroom so he didn't see us laughing. We clung together giggling. Not yet 5 and he's such a happy, charming chap. We do love him and it was wonderful seeing him do something so clever yet "normal".

Because that's what you yearn for when you are living with cancer, for the "normal" you want to return and the "abnormal", i.e. the cancer, to be gone.

Sadly, for both George and Mum, it wasn't.

CHAPTER SEVEN

The Absolute Pits: Part Two

June and July rushed on and, every day, it seemed there was something new and exciting which would distract us from the constant grind of having illness in the family.

The Queen's Diamond Jubilee was celebrated in rain. The Cricket, Ascot and Wimbledon kept us fascinated, particularly with poor Andy Murray getting so near and yet still being so far away from that record breaking moment when a Brit would finally win Wimbledon again. How I celebrated when he got the Gold at the Olympics and the make-believe champagne got cracked when he finally won the US Open at the end of the year. Roll on Wimbledon 2013 when I hope to open a bottle of the real stuff!

Richard and Shauna brought the twins over for a week-long visit. After the first initial "what the hell are these little things?" sniffing check out from Bonnie, she decided Sophia and Isabella were wonderful and never left them alone, probably because they, in turn, delighted in dropping food down to her and seeing how fast she could catch it.

Halfway through the week, Shauna finally solved the mystery of why Sophia always had one wet sock. She followed Bonnie into the kitchen to see what she was so interested in and found her eldest daughter hanging on to the work-surface, puddle jumping one foot into Bonnie's water bowl. We women only had one other tussle - to get the men away from the Olympics on television. When we did, we had a wonderful week enjoying normal, everyday things.

George kept going very well and almost managed to ignore his constant tiredness. He seemed on as good form as he had for a very long time.

And, for one brief while, I was the one doing the sympathising, not the one being sympathised over. My great friend, Theresa, who has been another constant source of strength and advice to me, was now facing similar anxiety about her family.

Friday 15th June

'Theresa rang this evening with news that her Mum has had a strangulated hernia whilst visiting her brother Anthony in America. Anthony had a suspected heart attack and then spinal problems only months ago and we agreed that what is happening to us all with multiple worries is unprecedented. She has a close friend with awful cancer too. Mum had her third chemo today, and I had actually forgotten she was due to have it. Can you believe that! I know you have to expect all this as you get older, but this is beyond comprehension. So much all at the same time! Compounding this, and never before seen, is this cold and wet spell in June. The weather has been mostly grey and miserable all day. I'm still in winter clothes, which is ridiculous. The world seems to be upside down.'

Whilst one great friend was worrying about her loved ones, my other great friend, Monty, who only lives around the corner from me, was enjoying a completely different time. She was having great fun choosing a new car. In May she had asked me to go with her to test drive a Fiat 500. Now, even she will admit, when it comes to cars, she doesn't have much of a clue.

"Why me? Why not one of your son-in-laws?"

"They're both up to their necks at work and you know loads about cars."

Believe me; I don't!

The test drive was an absolute hoot. Talk about the blind leading the blind! She couldn't make up her mind between a manual and an automatic. We took out the manual first. She asked the salesman to come with us. He convinced us we should take it out on our own. I knew we were in for fun when she couldn't even seem to see where any of the controls were.

"I don't like driving other people's cars," she protested.

"But this is a test run. You've got to try driving it," I encouraged her.

By the time we careered into one car park to try out how much room there was in the back seat, she was already convinced this was the car for her, but was it to be a manual or an automatic? Both have only two doors and I couldn't remember the last time I'd even tried to get into the back of a car so tiny. For some reason, I couldn't get my high heels, big bum and long legs in behind the folded down front seat. Monty was more agile. She managed to get in from the driver's side, but then couldn't get out again going forwards. I tried pushing her from the passenger side. She started laughing and flopped back into the seat.

"Try going out backwards," I suggested. "You got in that way."

It worked, but only after I gave her a damned good push. When we got back to the showroom, the salesman showed us that we'd only been bringing the front seats forward half way. Did we feel like fools when we saw how easy it was to push them out of the way if you pulled on the right levers!

When we took the automatic car to another car park for her to practise reversing, I was convinced that car also had parking sensors, as the manual before had, and she trusted me. This one didn't!

"That tree's getting bigger and bigger in my mirror," she said.

"Don't worry," I answered blithely. "The sensors'll start beeping in a mo."

There weren't any; so of course, they didn't.

She finally stopped. We got out and checked how close she'd got. You couldn't have got a tissue paper between the tree and the car. Shaken, but definitely not stirred, we exploded into fits of giggles. Other parkers must have looked at us and thought "what are those mad women up to?"

Her new baby arrived on 4th July and she was over the moon that the different sized poppy stickers she chose to decorate it with looked so good.   Needless to say, the car is also now called Poppy and I was the first one to be offered a lift in it.

It proved to be the last time I had a belly laugh and some on-going fun for ages.

A few days later, on a Sunday, Mum had problems with the pic line used for her chemo. When the District Nurse called to prepare her for her next chemo, she found that a nurse had failed to flush it out when she'd finished the last chemo and it had blocked. She would need a new line put in and that would, again, delay her next chemo session booked for the next day.

My 80 year old Mum was told it could be sorted out that Sunday but only if she could get herself to the hospital at Cheltenham. Because Worcester is a satellite unit of the main Oncology unit at Cheltenham, there was no cover there over the weekend. There was no one to drive her the 50 or so miles there and back. We agreed it was ludicrous. How can Doctors, like Mr Pandey, be expected to do all their magnificent work and then the back-up not be in place if something as simple and obvious as this goes wrong? The unit was all geared up for her to be there the next day. Now they were going to have to squeeze her in some time later and that was, surely, going to cost money. We talked long and hard about how un-cost effective it is to not have some back-up arrangements in place for weekends. It seems hospitals nowadays are trying to work only 9 to 5, Monday to Friday.

When I spouted off about the nurse not flushing out the pic line, Monty, who also used to be a nurse and has great sympathy for them, calmed me down saying what she'd said to me many times before. "Sadly, nurses aren't like we'd like them to be because they're under too much pressure."

In calmer moments, I know she's right. In recent years, to us, it's become more obvious just how unhappy nurses are. We hear them moaning all the time, but, sadly, they're doing it to the wrong people. It's no good moaning to the patients. Only management will ever sort anything out.

If I ran the NHS I'd start sorting out its messes by first looking at the role of nurses. Nurses are lynch pins. They are the glue which really makes hospitals work and I just don't understand why no one seems able to see that the role they are now being asked to undertake simply isn't working that well.

I would open up the nursing profession more. I'd bring back different types of nurses, those who keep patients clean, fed and comfortable and those who observe, monitor the drugs and administer patient's recovery – and I'd make sure all of them had adequate training

But more than anything, I'd look at changing the hospital routine, the timing of shifts and what happens when, particularly on the wards. There, I would start by firstly looking at when patients need rest and make sure they got enough of it by working the daily timetable around it. For example, waking patients up at 6.am for obs, then again at 8am for their breakfast gives the patient no chance to get proper rest. It's all designed around the staff shifts.

Wards are far too noisy nowadays. I would put ward nurses back on to the wards for most of their working hours to ensure that patients have everything they need to recover swiftly. I'd make sure nurses spend most of their time away from their computers and form filling so that they can do what they are trained to do – nurse patients.

Nurses aren't "angels" and we are wrong to expect them to be. They are human beings trained and willing to follow a rewarding career but they're being asked to do too much. Patients and their relatives always look to the nurse for reassurance. Nurses need to be allowed to get on and do what they do best. In the modern NHS, that simply isn't happening.

But, enough of my rants!

George was coming up to the date of his next CT Scan and he appeared to be doing so well, we'd taken our eye of the ball.

Wednesday 11th July

'Yay! We booked a holiday today. A direct flight to Lake Garda – Sept 9th. We just decided – and did it – and it felt so normal and good to be able to be spontaneous. I hope we actually take this holiday and nothing goes wrong.'

My friend Theresa's mother had recovered enough to travel home from America. She, too, lives a flight away from her parents and she'd been to see them to make sure they had everything they needed.

Saturday 14th July

'Speaking to Theresa and finding out how she found her parents has made me realise again that in spite of the pressure of all my problems, hers are actually no different. Distance is as much a problem for her as for me. Those miles apart are proving damned problematical as our parents age.'

For several months, George had been aware of a lump on his scalp which seemed to appear suddenly in the bald patch of his "monk's tonsure". He'd asked me to look at it. It didn't look that bad to me and we agreed that we would just keep an eye on it until he was due to see Ajay Kumar for a routine check-up on his kidney. Ajay, didn't seem too concerned, but arranged an x-ray to be on the safe side. After that, we were due to see Amanda Jones, so Ajay said she'd give us the results.

They weren't at all good:

Tuesday 14th August

'My dear, sweet, George is in the wars again.

Ajay Kumar thinks the lump on his scalp is renal cancer. Amanda Jones is concerned it may be nothing more than a cyst and it should be confirmed before she does anything further. Ajay and the radiographers think George needs radiation as soon as possible. A.J. would prefer to wait for a fine needle biopsy, but Dr Southall, the only pathologist who can do it, is away on holiday. Ajay has stopped G's Ciclosporin (anti-rejection drug) with immediate effect to try to encourage the body to fight the cancer. George will now need close monitoring to avoid rejection of the transplant. George has already said he never wants dialysis again. We have to allow the medical experts time to consider all options so they get the best outcome by giving the best treatment in the best order.

TIME! Oh God, time! How much time do we have? Can we wait this long now they have found something – but what have they found? Every bone in my body is saying we should get on and do something, anything...

I prayed two days ago for the pressure on us to be lifted. This is hardly an answer to my prayers, so now I shall have to go back to praying for G's healing and that they make the correct decision in enough time.'

It looked like we would have a two week wait before the fine needle aspiration could be carried out. It was an excruciating wait:

Wednesday 15th August

'The trouble with waiting periods like we are enduring is that they are energy sapping. It's almost a case of emotion suspended not emotion drained because you have to keep going and you daren't let yourself go. If you ever did you'd never be able to rein yourself back in.

I don't know what to think. I don't even know what to pray for. There are such severe downsides to all sides of the argument. The worst is seeing George so quiet.'

There was just no respite from the wait, but that didn't stop other things happening. Mum was coming to the end of her chemo and all she could talk about was coming to visit us in Jersey. Jim and I agreed they should wait before they booked anything, but no, she was adamant. She wanted to fly over sometime during the week before we were due to go to Lake Garda and to stay for a month.

"But we won't be there for your first week if you do that," I gently protested.

"Doesn't matter. Jim and I can look after Bonnie. We need a change of scenery."

There was no doubting that. Jim had been a tower of strength whilst she was having chemo and he needed a break if nothing else.

"But what happens if George has to go away for treatment as soon as we get back?"

"Then you'll definitely need someone to look after the dog. You're not putting her in kennels when we can look after her."

My Mum was on her own little mission and nothing Jim or I could say would stop her! And who would want to stop her after the ordeal she'd been going through all year. I am so proud of my Mum and her resilience. Bonnie rather enjoyed the arrangement too!

Koo, Steve and   were also due over for the August Bank Holiday week. We were both longing to see them but we had to get ready for them to visit. George had another CT scan unexpectedly. I was exhausted with all the extra work getting ready before they arrived and the thought of that week on Lake Garda was the only thing that was keeping me going.

Worse was to come.

Thursday 23 August

'Bring us your sick and needy. George and I rescued a hedgehog in the early hours. It had its nose stuck in a cottage cheese pot. I woke to hear it going around in circles banging its head against the cars in the drive. I made George get up. "Why?" he moaned. "Because you're the man in the family!" I snapped back. He wasn't best pleased. When we got downstairs it had disappeared. We caught up with it going up the road, me in my nightie, but at least George had his trousers on. He held the wee thing between his slippered feet as I pulled the pot off its nose, then the damn thing just sat there and looked up at us.

We had a terse discussion as to whether it would be best to pick it up and put it in the hedge or just let it get there after we'd gone. Neither of us had gloves on. We decided to leave it. As we walked away, looking back all the time, it took a few hesitant steps towards the hedge and then it turned right back into the middle of the road.

"It'll sort itself out." George had had enough. "And just look at what you're wearing."

My nightie was a bit skimpy! Thank God only the hedgehog was there to see it!

Walking back, we looked up at the most spectacular canopy of stars. It was so clear. George suddenly stopped and said "I've got a line all the way down my one eye."

Oh, what now!

We went back to bed, but I couldn't settle. I got up and rang A&E. By 5.45 am we were in there. A lovely young Doctor said there was something definitely there, but it was small. He suggested George saw his Optician that day so it could be compared to previous pictures of the eye.

Coming home at 6.15 am, we found the hedgehog we'd rescued flattened exactly where we'd left it in the road. Well, that was a waste of effort.

Later, I had lunch with Monty and got home to get an email from Ann saying the hedgehog probably was so shocked at seeing great, big, ugly, old me when the pot came off its face, it couldn't move! That's why it got run over. Charming!

Meanwhile, George spent 2 hours at the Opticians. He has a big floater, needs to see a specialist promptly, but they can't reach anyone at the hospital – they're all operating, so that has to be fitted in now too. Oh hell.

And then Monty rang this evening to say we'd caused a major search for her whilst we were out. What?! It seems she forgot she was supposed to be filling in at work instead of being with me and they were so worried as she never forgets anything, they sent the search parties out. Well, at least it proves she's loved.

I kept going until 9pm, then collapsed. It's been a bizarre, worrying, ludicrously funny, old day and now I'm just terribly tired.'

George finally got the last appointment of the day with the eye specialist for the following Tuesday 28th August, bang in the middle of Koo, Steve and Sam's visit. We tried to carry on as if there was nothing to worry about, but every now and then I caught Kirstie sticking very close to her Dad. She never once said how worried she was, and neither did I, but it was obvious the worry was hanging over all of us like a black cloud. Only Sam, at five years old, seemed oblivious, so we concentrated all our efforts on having fun with him.

It turned out George had a retinal tear, probably exacerbated by a fall he'd had the day before when he slipped down a step in our neighbour's garden when he'd gone round to water their plants for them. The Consultant opened up the eye clinic at the hospital and at 7pm he lasered the tear to mend it.

He even let me watch as he did it, but I have to admit it was all a bit boring.

Wednesday 29th August, George had a check-up with Ajay to check how he was doing after coming off the anti-rejection drug. All seemed well there, but, suspiciously, there were no results yet from the CT scan.

We should have guessed we were about to be given even more bad news.

CHAPTER EIGHT

Hopes and Desires

Friday 31st August

'The cancer has gone to George's brain, or so they assume.

There will now be more tests. George has been told about radiotherapy, more medicine, more chemotherapy.

He's been stopped from driving.

Suddenly our world has juddered to another halt.

I refuse to let his end of life be unhappy.

We'll do what we can.

Oh God; why are you being so cruel?'

The lump on the scalp was growing fast and, bizarrely, George was experiencing excruciating pain in his hip. Amanda Jones wanted to do another MRI and the hours until the urgent appointment was confirmed went by in a shocked blur. I experienced some of my lowest and blackest hours over that weekend. I hate to think what George was thinking, but this time we were just too shocked to even talk.

Monday 3rd September

'The tears came this morning for George who said he wants to go on holiday as he thinks it will be our last holiday together. They had to come. Mine flowed with his. This is just so bloody miserable.

BUT the MRI is tomorrow. Aviva are being very helpful, we see Amanda Jones Thursday, and perhaps, just perhaps, the waiting is over and we can get on with fighting this awful illness.

Bonnie gave both of us extra big licks when we went down to breakfast. Even she knew something was wrong and was very quiet and well behaved until she started coughing. We've heard that cough before and knew what it was. Sure enough, Bonnie has kennel cough, so it was an early afternoon visit to the Vets for an antibiotic jab and a vaccine up the nose for her. Afterwards I had tea with Monty and a bit of a chat where I literally collapsed with exhaustion but after a piece of coffee and walnut cake things looked better and I decided I'm not giving up just yet.'

Tuesday 4th September

'George had his MRI on the brain and X-ray of the hip today. Whilst I waited, I met Ajay who's deeply aware that George might lose his kidney. I'm worried sick about G dying. G is almost silent, but we have to keep reminding both him and me that he's not dead yet and he's doing as much now as he was three weeks ago. There's a strange sense of – what? - impossibility. I really do find it hard to believe all of this is true and I keep thinking something else is going to happen. Yet, I saw the scan with my very own eyes and the shadowing was very prominent. Perhaps I'm burying my head in the sand.'

Mum, too, was waiting for the results of her first scan after finishing chemotherapy.

Wednesday 5th September

'Partial relief. Mum's results show the bowel looking normal and the spots on her liver and kidney have reduced, thank God. She says she's feeling much better.'

The relief didn't last...

Thursday 6th September

'Well, God has deserted us. There are now three spots of cancer in the brain, in different parts, still small, so they will have to do even more radiotherapy/Sunitinib. My hardest part is that George looks so well, it's hard to accept he could well lose this fight. George finally asked THE question and Amanda Jones is saying 18 months is a reasonable time frame, but who knows? I'm angry, sad, stunned, disbelieving, all at the same time - and all at sea. So, no matter what happens I will try to make our final time together as happy as it can be.'

… but the sense of total bewilderment did.

Amanda Jones said it would probably take a good week for her to arrange the radiotherapy in Southampton and all the other appointments we would need following that, so whilst she was doing that we should go on holiday and have a good time.

Friday 7th September

'This is truly bizarre. We were given no doubt yesterday that George could die, but today it's as if absolutely nothing is happening. A busy day getting ready to go on holiday – perhaps this is how you handle it.'

On top of everything, my Mum, who I dearly wanted to see, was due to arrive for her visit but the only flight I could get for her and Jim landed twelve hours before we were due to depart. I felt incredibly guilty. My Mum arrived like a whirlwind, full of vim and vigour, and told me we must go.

Saturday 9th September

'Well, Mum's here, exactly the same apart from her poor hair, cropped and frizzy, but other than that there's nothing to show she's just come off chemotherapy. Jim's a treasure; looks after her amazingly. Within minutes of watching the suitcases being unpacked, Bonnie completely abandoned us and is now following my mother everywhere. Talk about cupboard love! I wish we weren't going on holiday tomorrow, but I appreciate that we need that too and I'm actually quite excited. I hope it all goes well. '

It did – and it proved to be exactly the week we needed together to come to terms with what was going to happen next – and really, just to celebrate our love for one another. Whilst I was there on Lake Garda, I was able to express all the pent up emotions I was feeling – and George certainly appreciated the chance to just be together, alone, too. We needed it to be a special time, without worries, but life and all its inconveniences goes on regardless of how unwell you are.

Sunday 9th September

'5am start and we started in such good spirits. The direct flight to Verona was easy, the drive to Lake Garda got prettier and prettier; then Riva del Garda was exactly what we needed.

Then down to earth with a bump. The room at the Hotel Sole overlooked the kitchens. We'd booked- and paid a lot of money for - a Lake view. George was devastated. We complained. They protested they were fully booked. George crumpled. I had to go into action. I threatened moving to a five star at €800 per night! It was the fault of the tour operator who hadn't sent on the request, not the hotel, but the hotel responded brilliantly and we got our Lake view which I am looking at now.

It is exactly what we need and from there on the day just got better. It's lovely.'

George has never had any trouble talking about his cancer, and has often jokingly described the cancer cells either as his P.L.C. = pesky little critter, or his "unwanted lodgers". Now, he started referring to his "lodgers" all the time and seemed unable to say the word "cancer".

Monday 10th September

It's odd that I started to write May instead of September. On the surface, I'm calm, but underneath I'm a wreck. We came to bed this evening, George had had too much to drink, and he started talking about his "lodgers" with that bravery that takes my breath away and makes my heart beat more heavily, so heavy it's like a tonne weight in my chest.

He has to talk. I have to talk too; but what we are talking about has such limitations. We know he has lesions on the brain from this persistently evil cancer; we know he will have radiotherapy/ chemotherapy when get back, but after that what do we know?

We've heard all they've said about brain power loss, that the Sunitinib will only retain its use for around 18 months, but as we talk, what are we actually talking about? Our worries? Not really. Matters are settled as much as we can have them at this point.

Our love for each other? That grows deeper as each day takes us another step towards being parted. The more we talk about it, the more we somehow trivialise what is actually a grand passion and strength, so strong no-one has ever been able to rattle it.

We talk about the children, how we love them and are proud of the lives they're making for themselves; how their children are wonderful and what good parents they are to them. We worry about the hardships they face, but they are (pretty much) fit, healthy and happy. We had to live our lives with far harder choices to make and <u>many</u> more horrible problems to overcome.

So really, provided the children can continue going on as they are, we believe they will be okay.

So, that leaves us with nothing to talk about which is fresh. We go over the same things time and again. We look at the beautiful Lake Garda view we fought so hard to get – I even complained to a very hard-nosed rep today and managed to get the better of her – but I got no satisfaction from it. Yesterday, no view, I fought, we got and I felt better. Today, I fought and I felt embarrassed. It's not worth doing. Why is nothing ever easy, particularly when we have so much to face when we go back?

A ferry trip to Limone was very successful but reassured us we'd done the right thing coming to much more spacious Riva, which is also flat. As I watch the sparkling lights late at night on this quiet Lake, I know that for certain.'

Tuesday 11th September

'It's been a lovely day, sunny. We went to Malcesine and were surprised at its size. George didn't complain once as we shopped – must be these new pills he's on because he's certainly walking further and more energetically and he's hardly complaining about aches and pains.

As I write, he's sitting at the window overlooking the Lake, reading. I find it amazing that he's so unruffled considering the news got worse by the minute last week and he's facing such horrendous treatment. All he will say is "there's nothing I can do. I've got it. It's my illness, but they're offering help and I'm going to take it," and it's true; he needs to accept what's on offer at this point.

So after coming back to Riva, we sat on the harbour wall eating Amaretto and Frutti di Bosco yoghurt ice creams, feeding each other and giggling like kids.

On the boat, we'd celebrated with two Scots ladies Andy Murray's win at the US Open (his first Grand Slam) and now we're about to head for dinner where we'll order something special to drink. Heaven is here in this little part of the Dolomites.

And I have one, irrational, wish. I see George's "unwanted lodgers" as being unhappy because they can only destroy and never build anything for themselves. I wish we could leave them here in the Dolomites where amongst its beauty they could find their own form of contentment and stop trying to ruin ours. They are unwelcome with us in Jersey.'

Wednesday 12th September

"This morning Verona, this afternoon back to Riva "...I keep singing that song from Kiss Me Kate – what is it? "We opened in …." And ends " …and there we are, de-dum-di-da, something, something, back in Padua…"

Verona was lovely and sunny. Thomas, the Danish flirt of a courier, made us laugh all the way down through vineyards: Bardolino, Veneto, lovely, lovely countryside on the Achige River bounded by those verdant, white rock formations which stick up like a hedgehog's needles, consistent only in that after one you can always see another two or three, side sloping, needle topped.

Thomas stunned me. He was probably late 30s, slim, attractive, but so much younger than me. At Juliet's Balcony, better than I expected but not half as interesting as other older and more ornate balconies we saw further back in the old town, we asked Thomas where we could buy another dress to go with the one we bought the twins yesterday in Malcesine. I told him I'd lived for a while in Denmark and had gone to school there, but I couldn't recall a word of the Danish I'd learned, to which he replied "Jeg Eskede Dag". I was so stunned to have a young, attractive man flirt with me; I turned to George and said "this young man has just told me he loves me." Thomas had the grace to blush.

This holiday is doing me good!!

It's late afternoon and the promised rain is teaming down spectacularly. The Lake views have all but disappeared as we look out of the window. George reads and I shall write more here where heaven sits amongst the raindrops leaving me relaxed when I should be worrying.'

?Thursday ?13th September

'See. I don't even know what day it is. This place has put a spell on me and in spite of the awfulness of what we have to go home to, I've relaxed, I'm thoroughly enjoying myself and things are amusing and entertaining me.

My day of "attractiveness" continued on into the evening. We walked into dinner and the trainee wine waiter, who must be all of 18, and who had got all confused when he said "when are you", not "how are you" at breakfast, gave me the cheekiest, boldly flirtatious, wink. George guffawed, but he changed his tune later that evening when the most elegant of the 'outdoor' waiters seemed to take a shine to me. "He's only after a big tip," I protested, actually enjoying the attention. "Phaw! If that's what you think", I got back from George. Whatever, it was, I was very pleased to be reminded I could still attract some attention. This illness has made me feel old and haggard,

I came back down to earth when the waiter told us he has a much younger, Brazilian, wife and that they are taking their son to Brazil at the end of the season to live there permanently because "Italy has nothing left". It's sad. This financial crisis is apparent everywhere.

So, late at night, I'm sitting with my notepad on my knees thinking how universal these financial problems are and how there is no getting away from them. George is again reading overlooking the Lake. God, how I wish I could take that window and its view home with us. It would be such an asset as he starts this ghastly treatment which makes him lose his hair, impairs his mind and isn't guaranteed to work. But as he says, he has no choice, so what else does he do?

And amongst such beauty, my tears did flow when I was alone in a toilet at Torbole today. We'd had the most delicious lunch and as I thought "Why can't it be like this every day?" I choked up and bolted for the Ladies. But these feelings are short lived and I refuse to let George see me cry. As the return to Jersey is approaching, I'm now torn between wanting to be home and getting on with it and dreading Sunday when we leave.'

Friday 14th September

'I've just showered after coming back from an all day trip into the Dolomites, which was easy, with spectacular light all day and just so relaxing.

The highlight came for me mid-afternoon when we went into part of the Adamello Brenta Geopark, to a valley with the Nordis Waterfall. We've taken some fantastic photos there and as we sat looking through them, I found myself praying that, here, George's "lodgers" would leave his brain to find a good home and that the fresh, clean water falling before our eyes would metaphysically wash over him and bring him back into full health.

If good can ever come from bad, on a day like this, in a place like that, then it has its very best chance.'

Saturday 15th September

'This morning, I noticed our toothbrushes in the bathroom. That's what I love about George. On holiday he always lays our toothbrushes alongside each other on his toothbrush holder. He always puts mine to the front. He's ever the gentleman. That's why I love him so much. He's so caring.

I'm writing this looking out over the view again. It's more noticeable at this time of the evening – sunset –but when the grey and white Dolostone and Limestone mountains take on a pink hue, the shape of a face appears at the top of the first pointed peak coming down towards the tiny village of Novene which twinkles its lights back at us all the way through the night.

The face looks like a Zephyr, or even a baby George, rather chubby cheeked with a high, intelligent forehead, placid, protecting. It's a perfect place for George's "lodgers" to live in perpetuity – they would be happy there looking always at the rich valleys at the feet of the Dolomites below them. So I said another little prayer begging for them to leave George's body and to re-locate there. They could watch the passegiate of Riva and Torbole; enjoy the Torbole big rock, which looks so like an ocean going liner moored close to the shore. They could watch the diners in the evening in the part ruined castle that the Hapsburgs built and which General Vendôme blew down with his one little cannon.

So much of the story of this region is slightly comic. The brown bears, Urse Brune, re-introduced with a gift of four Transylvanian bears have now multiplied to 32. A while ago one went walk-about into Bavaria. They wear radio tags, so it was daily news that the bear had gone on his holidays. There was much Italian discussion as to how they would coax him back home – food only partially worked. They decided to obtain a tranquilising shot and after tracking him down, decided on a day and a place to shoot it at him, load him on a lorry and bring him home. But before they did, some Bavarian bully hunted him down and shot him dead – and then kept the body. Discussions are on-going for his return.

On the trip down to Verona, the side of the roads have an odd, green, plastic sheet fencing, about 2 feet tall. There's a huge initiative going on to stop the local frogs from getting squashed on the busy road. They're trying to get to the river below to mate. Apparently, there has been so much road kill the road becomes slippery and treacherous. So, the fence, at great expense, was erected. The problem is, that even though they built overpasses and underpasses for the frogs, roe deer, snakes, etc. to get from the high slopes to the valley below, they forgot animals don't understand human bridges – nor can they read the signs in either of the two languages they put onto the fencing. The road kill continues.

Apparently, it's a constant source of discussion and moaning for the locals – and if the story didn't tickle me so much, I'd say "what were the idiots thinking! No wonder people moan!", but that's what irritates me most at the moment. I cannot stand to hear moaning, and I don't want to think about it. I want to scream "put up and shut up", when I hear any slight complaint. There are so many more important things to concentrate on – like George's illness.

George could moan. He certainly has reason to moan. But he won't. God knows how many medical staff have had to help him so far, so unless it is absolutely necessary he will never moan even to them how low he feels. But I've sat with him so often where staff treating him – particularly the nurses – have talked non-stop about themselves and what's wrong in their lives. Don't they understand that patients just don't want to hear it! Patients are battling their own worries and what they need is efficiency, allied to calm and polite behaviour, so when I see a nurse with hair flopping, too much make-up, or worse body piercings or tattoos, rushing around doing very little and moaning, moaning, moaning, my heart sinks. They're not happy and they don't seem to want their patients to be either.

But there I go – moaning – and apart from letting off steam, where is this rant going to get me?

I'd rather concentrate on the gorgeous day we've had again, a boat ride to Limone, a sit on the harbour, then a lunch of scallops and peaches followed by the most scrummy chocolate fondant. Superb but so simple.'

The holiday could not have been more timely. We got home on the Sunday and on the Monday, all the appointment letters arrived – to Southampton for the day on Thursday for the face mould to be made, back Monday to Friday the following week for radiotherapy.

The treatment had started.

CHAPTER NINE

Preparing For The Inevitable

Renal cancer is incurable. George has now lived with it for at least ten years, possibly longer. The native kidney in which the primary tumour was sited was found and removed in July 2003 but had been growing for a long time before. Luckily, after that, we did have nearly five years respite when we were able to live life to the fullest. The cancer revealed its slowly developing, unremitting, presence again in December 2008. We were warned then that that could be the end, but against all expectations we had got to August 2012 and found ourselves enjoying what looked like a quiet patch with the cancer slumbering.

But renal cancer only slumbers. It doesn't go away. September 2012 and we were back in the thick of it.

Wednesday 19th September

'It's a misapprehension when living with cancer that the patient "wants to talk". What they actually want to do is ignore the cancer and if they do need to talk they need to find a place or people who "make it comfortable for them to talk" because there comes a point where it is almost an embarrassment to admit that they still have cancer and aren't cured of it.

So that's what our good friends do. They allow us to talk and they listen without advising us too much. They know, as much as we ever can be, that we are now the experts. But the truth is; neither of us wants to be even that. George has found now, after all this time, that he needs enough information so he can get on with living with this illness, but not so much that there's no room for anything else in his life "to get in".

And then he simply wants to forget it and let his treatment and healing work as he enjoys his day to day life.

How do you do that with such a blackness enveloping you? The pain, physically, can be bad enough, but the pain, mentally, is harder.

George does it by being practical. He has his affairs in order and he keeps a close check on them. He makes sure he eats and drinks at regular times – and well. He does a certain amount of exercise by walking the dog. He reads the side effect warnings on his drugs and gets advice about it.

He tries to enhance the professional treatment by accepting it.

That's probably because, much as he'd like to, he cannot ignore that he has this horrible illness. It needs managing.

And ACCEPTANCE seems to be THE important part of keeping fighting this terrifying illness.

He has two main responses to the horror and fear we see in other people's faces when they realise he has a cancer which cannot be cured.

1) "Mustn't grumble" – because, as he says, there's no point.

2) "Get on with it".

Which is why he calls the renal cancer which spreads like a dandelion clock spread in the wind, the "PLC" (pesky little critter) and the lesions in his body "the lodgers". He is in no doubt at all that he wants those unwanted lodgers evicted.

He has to go through all-head radiotherapy next week to have half a chance. After that, he has to go back on Sunitinib with all its uncomfortable side effects because a) they know it works for him and b) there's very little else on the market they know and trust.

There's that word again – TRUST – but with trust we've had nine years together we so well might never have had and I, certainly, trust that there will be many more days making many more months and hopefully making many more years in which we can cuddle and laugh and above all _love_.'

It wasn't all satisfactory. With going on holiday and then the treatment days in Southampton, the twenty eight days I could have spent with Mum and Jim came down to fourteen.

I'd wanted to spoil my Mum, to take care of her, and she ended up taking care of George and me. At times she took over the cooking and cleaning and certainly Bonnie made sure she took over care of her. Bonnie is devoted to my mother (could be something to do with the treats she gets!) so I was happy that at least she was getting some decent fussing. I coped, and managed to enjoy my limited time with Mum and Jim. People even told me I was looking well, but I knew my stress levels were through the ceiling.

Friday 21st September

I couldn't write in here last night. It was such a big day which ended up a bit of a turning point.

We set off to Southampton for the day yesterday so the radiotherapy mask could be made. On the 10am plane, which had Mary Peters the Olympian plastered on the side to celebrate the Olympics, I sat in 17A alongside the window. For ten minutes, before take-off, I watched the ground crew and pilot check the wheel undercarriage right below me. They were obviously assessing damage.

All I could think was "well, if this plane crashes, I hope we go together". When we talked about it when we got back on the same plane to return later in the day, George confirmed he had been thinking the same as well and that "this could be the easy way out".

I keep thinking about how dogs in pain deliberately go out into the traffic to put an end to their agony. A human's not allowed to do that. They're expected to be brave and to endure the most unpleasant of treatments.

And I ask myself "why?"

In fact yesterday went quicker and smoother than we expected. We arrived three hours early for the appointment, but they were able to see us straight away.

I watched as George's radiation face mask was made, a blue plastic thing which holds him absolutely still. I listened to the Consultant, lovely Charles Hamilton, as he explained what to expect – was most encouraged when he told us how robust the brain is for this kind of treatment, then my heart dipped and rallied as he said it's 50/50 whether it's successful.

He says there should not be any personality change, but surely he means from the treatment. He can't possibly predict what the illness is going to do, can he?'

Information specific to your case always comes new to you and is delivered by the professionals, usually, explaining the best and worst scenarios. You know you have to listen to what the experts say, but there's always that damned niggle in the back of your mind caused by the snatches of information you've picked up along the course of your life, some right, some wrong, some real, some fictional. Every stage of cancer treatment requires a steep, uphill learning curve for both patient and family.

At times, I've floundered and been overwhelmed. I've also found it damned hard to ignore everything I've heard before and, and at times it's been easier to cling on to what a good friend has said rather than the words of a stranger, no matter how expert they were. I've been so desperate for comfort.

Then, there's the other side. It's hard to remember you, and the patient, sadly, are not the only people fighting cancer. Cancer is everywhere and many other people have to deal with it too. You must never forget that.

My good friend, Monty, lost her husband to cancer ten years ago but she never fails to ask us how things are going. I'm comfortable talking to her, but every now and then, I wonder at what cost to her own sense of loss she's talking to me.

It was her birthday the day we went to Southampton for the face mask to be made.

Friday 21st September – continued

'So, I rang Monty to wish her Happy Birthday. She wanted to know what happened, so I told her, trying always to be positive. But it brought back to her how Richard had rallied on Dexamethasone although it was already too late for his secondarys to be treated. It's 10 years since he died. I wonder whether I should talk so openly to Monty and if she finds talking about it still sore. She says she's used to being a widow now, but there are obviously still times when Richard's passing away is hard to deal with. Am I asking too much of my friend?'

That was another weekend that was hard to deal with.

Saturday 22nd September

'Have I woken up angry! As I write, I can hardly hold the pen and make it go where I want it to. My handwriting is a random scrawl.

I went to bed with a tummy ache. My stomach and chest have been tense (along with my jaw) for weeks now and I'm obsessed with having regular bowel movements in the hope they make me feel better.

I woke dreaming of a shit covered toilet that I couldn't clean. I kept trying everything that I could think of to make it go away, but it was impossible.

George was already awake but tense. Bonnie yapped and bounced around in the car as I drove to Noirmont for her walk. I got stuck behind a doddery old lady in a Polo doing 23 mph and then George lost his temper when I gave way to let a white van get past the parked cars half way down that road.

Mum had already urged me to pick up Bonnie's poo from the garden, which I'd obediently done. She and Jim shouldn't be doing that! But by the time I'd parked the car Bonnie had trampled all over the bag we took with us to put in the poo bin and the crap was in the back of the car.

I lost it and screamed at her. George lost it and snapped at me. And for once I screamed back at him, so he smashed her ball thrower and broke it, declared "I want to die" and stormed back towards the car.

"You'll need these then." I threw the car keys after him. "And your walking stick."

At that point, even he realised he'd gone off like a train without it. We looked at each other as if to say "oh, bugger" and continued the walk. He cuddled me half way round. I said "I refuse to say sorry. I'm not sorry. I needed that".

He knows how stressed I am and that he mustn't always expect to lean on me, but as he has to so many times, he always tries to ask me nicely. He knows I'm not superwoman.

Back at home, we were back to normal with each other, but my Mum had suddenly developed a wobbly.

Thank God for the vacuum cleaner and the iron. I sorted her out and then bashed hell out of them!

When there's nothing wrong with anyone, you could have a full blown row. With this ghastly cancer, you are always on tenterhooks not to upset the sufferer more. At this precise moment, I don't know who to feel most sorry for – me, who never asked to be caught up in all of this, or Mum and George – who definitely never wanted to have it.

George says being the carer is worse. The patient has the right to feel all the emotions that go with the illness. The poor carer just has to wait and watch and react, while putting their own life onto a different course to what they expected. Quite often, they have to put their own life on hold.

I just think any crisis creates change. You just have to deal with it. Today, I've dealt with it my losing my temper and I feel better now.'

I had a patch of talking to myself at that point. No matter what I was physically doing, I found myself muttering to myself "I am so fed up!" It had to stop. I was driving myself mad. So in the middle of yet another sleep disturbed night I decided I had to change my thinking. "Fed Up" had to be replaced by something. I decided on:

Forget

Everything (that's happened)

Don't

Underestimate

Positive thinking.

Living with cancer in the family never changes your personality, but it plays havoc with your emotions. It may change your routine, your rhythm in life, your outlook, but it won't change who you are essentially.

We've always tried to avoid becoming cancer "bores" because being one can be so off-putting, but when you have little else on your mind, it can be very hard to find anything else to talk about. You have so little time for anything else.

So, long term illness can change your relationship with other people. There is the old saying "a friend in need is a friend indeed." At times of illness, the "friends" you expect to be there for you, aren't always. Some people can deal with illness. Others simply can't. Some people love gossiping about it and the gorier your ailment, the more relish they seem to savour. Others start to avoid you. They simply don't know what to say to you. You have to respect all reactions, particularly if the person chooses to be honest with you.

The trouble is, that doesn't stop their reaction to your cancer hurting.

Monday 1st October

'The backlash has started. People can only maintain sympathy for so long. Good friends do it for ever, but there will always be some who resent you

for taking centre stage, or, more stupidly, upstaging them by being ill. George and I try to only talk about what we're going through if pushed. We've become quite adept at changing the subject because we're more bored with what we're having to put up with than they will ever be, but there's always one you can't deal with.

I had one today. ****** rang to see how we are getting on now we're back. She's diligent in keeping in touch, but we both know she's making a supreme effort. She wants to visit for coffee and I got the "no food though. I'm on a diet for my holiday. Then, I suppose I don't have to say that to you because you must be having to be very careful."

"What do you mean?"

"Well, it must be hard keeping to your diet, when George is so ill."

"Sorry? Do you mean I should be on a diet?"

"Well, you said you comfort eat when you're stressed. But, then, you're always stressed."

I thought I was handling it well, keeping my own thoughts to myself and to my writing diary. I obviously wasn't doing as well as I thought.

I heard myself say: "Well, would you like to be me at the moment?"

And I got back: "Everyone has things going wrong in their lives. You just have it all the time."

I actually felt guilty!! Then, I thought about it again and realised, sadly, not everyone has had the threat of death hanging over them for as long as George has. It has been going on a long time. It is boring.

Perhaps she was just having a bad day, but if she was, there's nothing I can do about it unless she tells me why. I was really pleased when she rang; not so pleased when I put the phone down. I sometimes wonder if people think we're making everything up that George has had to go through when he has survived, not died. He does never complain and most of the time doesn't look that unwell.

But, the truth is, he's been wonderful surviving everything he's had to put up with so far.

I stopped feeling guilty.

At the end of the day, it's her problem. Not mine. And when she comes, I shall offer her a whole, new, enormous, box of biscuits to go with her coffee. I bet she has two!'

The very next day we were invited to our other friends, Kath and Andrew, for afternoon tea. Spending time with them made me forget our other friend, but, when I think about it, I don't think I was fooling anyone trying to hide what I was actually feeling. They were just being wonderful friends going along with me and quietly supporting me.

Tuesday 2nd October

'A morning of chores, tea and good chat with Kath and Andrew, then an evening of better than usual TV.

But, I can still neither shake this general sense of resounding fatigue, nor the bitter taste of bewilderment hanging over me, though after yesterday's contretemps, I am trying to for everyone else's sake. I just can't stop seeing cancer everywhere.

Dear God, it is everywhere – brave stories in the newspapers, romanticised and dramatised in TV programmes, always a story or two doing the rounds about new wonder drugs which will give a few more months of life.

Do you avert your eyes and ignore all of them? I think, perhaps, it's best if you can.

The only true information you can trust is what the medical professionals give you. Then you trust your own gut reaction and intuition to that information.

After all, it remains your life, and the responsibility remains with you to make of that life what you can. As much as I love George and want to support him, only he can decide what he wants to do.

I am dreading George going back onto Sunitinib. I think it reduces his quality of life, but really it's not my decision. George is still perfectly capable of making his own mind up and as long as I see that, I have no right to affect his decision. He's preparing himself to go back on it, he wants to stay alive and I will do everything I can to help him. I'm just back peddling like fury to keep things as normal as I can for him.'

Throughout it all, George and I have relied on the children to keep us distracted with news of the grandchildren. Sam, aged five, had just started his second year at school and was battling the dreaded reading and writing. He's a bright little boy, very lively and chatty and we imagined he'd have trouble concentrating. With each telephone call came an update. He started slowly, then started to get the hang of things.   The first time he got ten out of ten for his spelling, there were celebrations all round.   Phew – another hurdle passed.

Then came exciting news about the twins which took away the pain of rejection for me.

Thursday 4th October

'Another "Thank you but no thank you" on a spec piece of writing this morning – Oh well. That's part of a writer's life – rejection!

But, hey, why so grumpy? It is the most beautiful day and the news that Sophia and Isabella are in the new Cow & Gate advert (Supergroup) starting next week and despite Mum's sugar now being all over the place (bet she's been overdoing it now she's off the chemo), life's really not that bad. It's all a matter of perspective.

And talking of perspective, Richard rang this evening. Koo's taken the latest news about G's cancer badly but has been covering it up. Isn't that just Koo? George will have to do a lot of comforting, but quite how, I don't know. She's so capable as a wife and mother but every so often she still confounds us. Most of the time she's happy-go-lucky, but when something frightens her, she really can take it badly. If she were a horse she'd be a highly strung thoroughbred who spooks easily. Richard, on the other hand, gives the impression of being more grounded, but we know of old how deeply he hides things. George just wants Koo and Rich to be as close as possible and to be there for each other. When he's gone, he wants them to remain as close as they were as children.'

The time came for Mum and Jim to go back to their own home. George had suffered only a little irritation to his skin from the radiation up until then, but unseasonably warm weather was now giving him hell. I'd already anticipated what he would opt to do and on Thursday 4th October, I'd cut off a lock of his beautiful hair which was still as black as it had been when we were younger. I stuck it into my diary.

As soon as Mum and Jim had gone, he got me to take him to the Barber.

Monday 8th October

'George had all his hair shaved off this morning. I expected to be saddened, but in fact he has a lovely shaped head, which without hair shows off *his chubby apple cheeks and his smile. It's spoiled only by the tumorous bump. I wonder how long it will be before it grows back. No one's yet told us that. The poor girl in the Barbers was watery eyed as she was doing it.'*

The radiotherapy treatment was obviously working. The shaved head had raspberry blotches all over to prove it. Aqueous cream was used abundantly.

Tuesday 9th October

'Part of me wants to scoop George into my arms and cuddle him, but the rational side of me sees he's becoming increasingly sore and uncomfortable all over as a result of the radiotherapy, so I must hold back. Otherwise, I'm amazed how well he seems. Dr Hamilton did say he'd have few side effects. The main one seems to be the radiation burns, which are certainly obvious with increased redness, blistering and pimples. We were also told to expect a change in mood, though not personality, and fatigue. He is tired in odd ways, the most unusual for him being irrational short temper.'

The change went on for several days and then George was back to his usual self. I wondered what other people in the same position had to put up with and whether this very short reaction from George was due to his placid personality. He complained for a long time afterwards that his head felt "muzzy", but nothing worse.

Wednesday 10th October

'You can't predict cancer. It's a slippery eel which demands you track it as it goes through its onslaught on the ebb and flow of calmer waters. You just do not know what Cancer's going to do next, or how you are going to react to it, you just know it will do something you don't expect. Perhaps that's why it's so hard to evict the unwanted lodgers.'

That was the start of the last week of George being pretty well. He started back on the targeted chemotherapy Tuesday 16th October. This is what I wrote the next day when the weather had turned particularly nasty.

Wednesday 17ᵗʰ October

'*Two days of chemo and already George is not particularly well. I had a great time, but he's struggled through dinner with Dave and Julie this evening, so was glad to get home. We did have flu jabs yesterday. Perhaps that's contributing.*

The journey home was interesting. It's the highest tide of the year tonight. The Avenue was flooded and Beaumont was wheel high in water and seaweed. We avoided St Aubins and went up Beaumont Hill heading for higher ground. 25 years ago today the Great Hurricane hit. I hope we never see that again, nor what George is experiencing. I'm sad to see George go down so quickly with the side effects this time. I hate seeing him so washed out.'

We didn't know it, but we were about to be overtaken by another set of unexpected events.

CHAPTER TEN

And -Again!-We Get On With Living With Cancer

Bonnie is George's dog; always has been. Probably because of her sense of smell, within days of George starting chemo again, she was being extra careful around him. She's eight years old now, black as the night with a fast greying muzzle and white paws which look as though she's dipped them in a pot of white paint. She's a cross between a Labrador and a Collie, but though she looks – and eats! – like a Lab she has the Collie caring, watchful nature. Wherever George is, you can be sure to find Bonnie somewhere close.

In October, something odd started happening. Since she was a puppy, every evening after our meal, it's been her routine for her to bring a toy for me to play with her. It's the only time she ever shows me any real attention. I'm obviously nothing more than the cleaner and playmate in our family. She likes tug and rough and tumble, or chase and seek; anything energetic. Now, she started herding me towards a seat on the settee and would only let me have the toy when I was sitting in one corner.

Then she started jumping up next to me and continuing the game. As the days went on she started creeping onto my lap. She has never been a dog who likes to be fussed, or stroked, particularly by me. She's a very private dog, preferring her mat by George's chair. I have never been able to tickle her tummy.

Suddenly she was letting me stroke her. After a few days she would roll over and let me gently stroke her tummy. I thought at first she was trying to comfort me – and that really worried me. Why was she trying to comfort me?

And then I realised. She hadn't suddenly developed cancer. She must have had it for a very long time. She'd avoided being stroked because her skin was sore and sensitive.

When I asked Lindsey, the Vet, she agreed. "Is this a sign she's feeling better?" I asked.

"Could be, but we'll never really know. That's the trouble with cancer. We don't always know they've got it. If that cancer's been there for a long time, possibly even from birth, she will have been very careful to avoid being touched."

So, even the dog could have been living with cancer for up to eight years without it really showing. We'll just never know for sure.

Mum had a series of check-ups following on from the end of her chemotherapy. Mr Pandey, in her eyes still an object of grateful admiration, was pleased with her progress. He arranged regular scans to keep an eye on things. "He said I could have had it for years without any signs and without me knowing," she casually told me.

"Bowel cancer!" I was surprised. "Had you really never suspected anything?"

I thought back to signs I'd seen but hadn't thought to press her to follow up: swollen tummy, complaining about having to go to the toilet more frequently, not going at all. She's never made much an issue of them. Looking back, I think we'd all fallen into the trap of suspecting her diabetes and insulin dependency to be the probable cause.

"That's why it's such a beggar," Mum said. "It's bloody sneaky. It's really good at hiding and doing its damage. But most of it was my own fault. I thought I was just getting older and that's what happened when you got old. They can't do anything about ageing, can they? So I never really mentioned it. I suppose I should have."

That's another problem. If you don't talk about it, how is a Doctor ever going to know that there might be another problem?

Multiple ailments can be difficult to treat. The medication for one illness can cause problems in treating the other ailment. We've sat watching medical professionals weighing the benefits many times. But, where there is a concern, it must be discussed. It isn't time wasting. It can be a clue to something else going on. It's best to let the professionals – who have had the training – make the decisions.

And then it's up to the patient to follow their advice.

The end of October saw an upturn in everyone's spirits. Bonnie was better. My Mum was happy with how things were going. I'd had a really good run with my writing and had made some excellent new contacts. Bonzo had finished chemo and her hair was growing back. Even George seemed to be coping with the chemo despite having the dreaded side effects.

It helped this time that we had had previous experience, so we were more prepared. We had expected George to suffer side effects, so I'd stocked up on things that would help sooth them.

Nutrition is particularly important for the cancer patient. Chemo causes all kinds of side effects, but one of the most common is nausea and it's damned hard to keep eating when you are feeling sick. Making sure you follow a balanced diet is terribly important, and we knew from last time that George's taste buds were going to rapidly change. It was also terribly important for the health of his transplanted kidney that he maintained a good intake of fluids.

Instead of my usual style of cooking with spices and herbs, I'd learned then that I would need to revert to the same style of cooking as my grandmother had used – bland, lots of gravy, meat and two veg type meals.

Ajay Kumar had also told me last time to boost the amount of antioxidants George was getting from his diet by putting in as much fruit and veg as I could. Forget five a day. Ajay suggested eleven to thirteen was nearer the mark, but you try serving that much variety! Non-alcoholic cocktails became my speciality. Our favourite is pomegranate, blueberry and cranberry.

As with everything though, if you are diabetic you have to really watch the sugar content of fruit juices and tinned fruits. Specific dietary requirements must always be adhered to. Why make yourself ill when you are trying to make yourself better! So I never offered them to Mum.

I found the easiest dish for me to make was a pilaff into which you can throw all kinds of frozen vegetable. Mine's like a risotto but made with long grained rice. Stock cubes and herbs replaced more spicy flavouring. Dried oregano became a staple when even garlic became hard for George to take.

Meat dishes were no problem as long as they weren't highly seasoned. In came the good old shepherd's pie and out went the chilli con carne. George loves roasts and will happily eat cold meat as a leftover. He'll also eat game, so pheasant, partridge and pigeon were sometimes on the menu when I could get them. Boiled bacon and parsley sauce became a staple.

Out, though, sadly went fish. George and I love fish, but he just could not taste it, even if I made a fish pie. I can't stand macaroni cheese, but towards the end of the four week cycle, when George suffered terrible mouth ulcers, that was the thing George liked the most because it was soft.

That - and rice pudding. George got to the point where he couldn't even eat ice cream or yoghurt, but he never stopped eating rice pudding. To alter the monotony of rice pudding every day, I would add tinned peaches or – an absolute favourite which we've found is really good for calming down nausea – stewed apples. There is nothing like a good old Bramley Apple, stewed in a little sugar (or sugar substitute) to give that lovely old fashioned feeling of being satisfyingly full.

Tinned food – soups, stews, anything mushy - helped keep up George's calorie intake. Poached eggs, mini pork pies (the portions got smaller through the cycle) and prawns in watered down black bean sauce with lovely soft rice all helped to keep George eating when he really didn't feel like it.

Drinks became a problem too, but he knew he had to keep up his fluid intake to keep the transplanted kidney hydrated. So coffee and tea were served milky and so weak they looked like dishwater. Alcohol never tasted the same when he was taking the tablets, so wine and beer got replaced by stronger tasting organic cider or a tot of whisky every night "to sterilise the mouth".

I would watch George swill it round his mouth and grimace as the alcohol sparked up the ulcers. "Why are you even bothering?" I asked.

"Because it all feels so much better when it eventually goes down."

Bizarre! But, I don't question what he feels makes him more comfortable. Anything he can manage to consume is all right by me.

There is one recipe I make for George which I have to immediately warn isn't for everyone. A friend sent me a recipe from New Zealand reputed to have the great healing properties of Aloe Vera combined with Manuka Honey.

"BUT GET THIS ONE CHECKED OUT BY YOUR MEDICAL ADVISORS BEFORE YOU EVEN THINK ABOUT IT" came the warning in her email.

I did. Our Doctors were happy that we tried it. We call it "The Gunk" and certainly in soothing the soreness of the mouth, it worked for us.

Diabetics CAN NOT take this due to its high sugar content.

You need:

1lb of the best quality Manuka Honey you can afford, or, if not, a good quality honey.

4 leaves from the Aloe Vera plant

A tablespoon of whisky, brandy or rum – whichever suits your taste (as a preservative).

A sterilised bottle – the green or brown ones are best

To make:

Wash the Aloe Vera leaves and shave off the sharp edges. Cut into small pieces.

Liquidise these with the honey and whisky until smooth.

Strain into the sterilised bottle. Keep the bottle corked or with the screw cap on. The mixture will change colour from green to brown fairly quickly, so discard any which isn't used after four weeks.

Take one tablespoon a day before meals. Either, swill it around the mouth and then spit out, or:

It can be swallowed, but it can cause an upset stomach/diarrhoea, so be careful.

October passed into November. Koo and Sam came for a visit and we celebrated our 29th Wedding Anniversary with them at a local "Pirate Pete's". Little did I ever imagine that for our anniversary we'd go to one of these child friendly restaurants to celebrate. George could only manage a bowl of soup and an apple crumble, but Sam ate an enormous burger in between playing in the adventure room with friends he'd newly made.

After they went back, George was very lacklustre and our GP decided to take bloods. "Could be, you've just done too much," he said. "Get plenty of good rest. And be kind to yourself. You have got cancer, you know".

How could we forget! But, he obviously thought it important that George was reminded. It turned out he was right but not for that reason.

Thursday 8th November

'I should be going "grrrr" as I write because now George's healed ulcer site on his ankle – the one which caused so much pain and angst two years ago and which we've nursed religiously – is breaking down under the Sunitinib. Mo at Bethlehem (I love writing that, it's such a lovely thing to think you are going to a place called Bethlehem to visit the District Nurse dressing clinic) dressed it this morning and both of us felt relief Mo was still there so we didn't have to explain it all over again.'

The ulcer broke down quickly. George was being as stoic as ever but I could see he was in awful pain and the pressure of watching him suffer was starting to take its toll on me.

Saturday 10th November

'When did I start feeling ugly? It's sort of crept up on me without my noticing. Is it since G has had his renewed problems? Is worry making me ugly, or have I just stopped taking care of myself, so I feel ugly?'

You really have to take care of yourself as well as the patient. If the carer becomes ill, what happens then? Thinking back, I knew even then that we would need help – but both of us hate asking for it.

I know! It's irrational. You cannot expect to handle everything yourself. Help is there, but usually you have to be the one to initiate asking for it. Even when the help is offered, you find yourself saying "thanks, but we'll cope". It feels like pushing and pushing comes easy to some people but harder to others. For us, it comes really hard.

This time I had no choice but to ask for help. I was finding it difficult getting George in and out of bed; he was in so much pain. I rang the Palliative Team Leader of our local support organisation in Jersey, Family Nursing and Home Care.

"But, he's not dying," I caught myself reassuring myself.

"I know. But let's talk through who you need to talk to," she encouraged and in that one phone call I received not only an offer of practical help from her, but more importantly someone who could tell me what help was available and how I accessed it. She co-ordinated what I needed to do, in what order and offered to re-arrange appointments which we could no longer make.

Wednesday 14th November

'The ulcer is one goddamn awful mess and George is in the most tremendous pain with it. We had to call the Doctor in tonight and he immediately put George on morphine. This is happening fast. I don't like what I see.'

When crisis comes in cancer treatment, speed is essential. Infection can be fatal. By Sunday morning, I knew he needed to be in hospital – and fast.

Sunday 18th November

'G had to be admitted to hospital today. He woke in the most awful pain. I was going to ring the Doctor, then changed my mind and decided to ring Ajay instead. He's always said I could ring him any time, but I've never before had to. Luckily he was on weekend duty at the hospital. He told me what to do, even to getting George into the car and driving him myself as it would be quicker than sending out an ambulance. When I got there, they were at the door waiting for us and he was rushed up to the ward and put straight on an intravenous antibiotic.'

George had three different types of infection in the wound. If they hadn't acted as fast as they did, it could have been far more serious. His blood was already septic. He was seriously ill. He was in hospital for a week. I went into a state of suspended anticipation. On the surface I was functioning perfectly normally. Underneath, I was an absolute mess.

Tuesday 21st November

'As I write, I'm listening to the news. Palestinians in Gaza have 15 seconds to get shelter from Israel's bombing in retaliation to Hamas' constant pot-shotting into the disputed territories. Jeremy Bowen has just said "In Gaza violent death is seen as martyrdom."

Dear God, what are they thinking? That's not martyrdom; it's warfare with the innocents being used as cannon fodder. Do they really hold life so cheap?

It's all about damned power and retaining it. Headlining also is the news that Church of England Synod has bowed to vocal evangelists and voted against ordaining women Bishops. And these are believers in God, ergo the whole of humanity as I see it!! It beggars belief that they can ordain women as clerics, but then refuse them promotion. Will someone please tell me; what is the spiritual difference between a cleric and a Bishop other than a whole wallop of administrative duties and a fancier hat?

Okay, okay, their anger and muddled thinking is fuelling my anger. George's ulcer is worsening. A very nice nurse tonight could not put an adequate dressing on it. She was perfectly capable of sticking all sorts of needles into him, but she just did not know how to do something as basic as to get a wound dressing to stay on and make him more comfortable. He's in hospital, for God's sake! Aren't they supposed to be the experts!

But you daren't say anything. I'm keeping my mouth firmly shut in case they think I'm interfering. I got so wound up I screamed in fury as I drove out of the car park. Then, I got home and shrieked again in exhausted frustration. What else do we have put up with?'

Tension makes you see problems when there aren't any. An expert nurse later sorted out a regime for George's dressing and by the following Sunday he was able to come home. Getting George home was a relief even if he was terribly weak and needed a lot to be done for him.

Wednesday 5th December

'It took some arranging, but a whole bank of medical things got done and in a timely fashion. We've even had the podiatrist visit, so at least we've both now got happy feet.'

It was then I finally accepted we really needed everybody's help. I stopped trying to do everything myself, particularly when Mum's next scan showed spots on her liver and kidneys and that she would need more chemotherapy.

"Don't worry," she said. "You look after George and Jim will look after me. They've got my dates all sorted this time and anyway, if George can do it, I can do it, so will you please stop worrying. Oh, and did I tell you? I'm having a wig for Christmas. I'm fed up with this straggly old hair."

I listened to my wise old Mum. She told me emphatically that neither she nor George was giving up without a fight. They were both determined to get on with living with cancer.

When I broached this with George afterwards he said "well, what else do you expect us to do?"

Daily, I remind myself, neither are dead yet. Both have treatment to undergo, but there is treatment available and they are being offered it. We've been there before and, with help, we'll do it again.

Tuesday 11 December

'It's 29 years today since Granddad died. When I last sat with him, three weeks before he died, George and I had been married just three weeks. I showed him the photos and he said "I can go now you have someone to look after you." George has looked after me so well, but it's my turn now to look after the both of us until the time comes when I have to just look after myself. He's just gone to bed, exhausted. But the day has been so much better for him. We had a drive after the wound (improving) was dressed. We sat and had cake and coffee overlooking the harbour at St Aubins. It was such a lovely day. He seems happier and no longer confused from the infection. And Mum seems happier too. She got her wig today and she's really pleased with it. The battle continues, but we all seem to have had a rest day today. Here's to having many more of those rest days.'

Christmas was coming, but before that we had to see if the Mayan Long Calendar which predicted the end of the world on Friday 21st December 2012 was going to come true. In the back of my mind was the thought that it might be. We'd had such an awful year, it would seem right that everything ended in a big BOOM!

The day before, was a good day.

Thursday 20th December

'The MRI results show all three brain tumours appear to have shrunken. Mum had her line put in and her first chemo today. I should be jumping for joy – inside part of me is that we've passed yet another hurdle – but it's a restrained joy because there's still so much work to do.

BUT... As I write this this evening something is growing within me and I have a feeling it is renewed optimism. Both Mum and George have accepted and grasped what they have to do and if they can do it, then so can I.

If the world ends tomorrow, I shall die happy.'

Friday 21st December

'Well, the world didn't end today, but tonight, the heavens are crying as though it has. This rain is getting frightening.'

The news was pretty awful. Heavy rain had been falling for days and many people were flooded out. A storm hit Jersey and did a lot of damage. I was tired. I sat looking out of the window and made a momentous decision. I couldn't handle everything any more. I was going to have to give up work – to give up writing for a living.

And as I made that decision, by chance, my writing diary fell open at an entry I'd written on 30th September.

Sunday 30th September

'Full moon and October in only a few minutes. Where has the year gone!

No man should have a time put on his life – yet we humans do it all the time – you go to school for so many years, you shouldn't have sex before 16, you are expected to live perhaps so much time with cancer because that's what other patients have done before you. If that were true and it was all going to come together as an indication of the number of years we are predestined to live before we die, then that would give us all equal lives – and that's something we never have.

Which is what makes each day we live all the more important.

George has been tired and dull headed all day, but still managed to enjoy his lunch out with Anne and Alan. Now that is the essence of living life to the fullest. It isn't about the amount of experience you pack in or the things/money you achieve. It's about the quality and pleasure you derive from what you do and doing it with friends and family loving you is real living.

I never forget that quote from someone whose name I can never remember: "I have nothing to prove to anyone apart from myself".'

Life, for everything it is, was getting back to a new kind of normal as the year headed towards its close.

Monday 31st December

'I'll put this, my very last entry in this book and then I might do what I actually feel like doing - throwing the book in the rubbish. I would have preferred 2012 simply hadn't happened. It has been one long, uphill road with too many precipitous and blind corners. I can't imagine what 2013 will be like. 2013! Even the 13 sounds ominous.

It was another day much like yesterday. A slow start for George, a tiring trip to Bethlehem to get the wound dressed. I thought it would be a wash out of a day all round, but this evening I cheered up a bit when we watched a film called Secretariat about a racehorse who has never been beaten since the 1940s for holding the record of the 3 big American wins consecutively. I like films about beating the odds!

But strangely, I'm not downhearted. I've kept going all day. I feel released now I've turned my back on trying to sell my writing. It's taken the pressure off. From now on, I shall just write for myself and enjoy it for a while.

If I have one resolution for tomorrow, it will be that I refuse to have my own life taken away from me by this awful thing called cancer. I will continue to make my own choices when I am offered them.

And I will do everything in my power to help George, and Mum and Bonnie live as long as they can with the dreadful illness which is the killer cancer, but which we know so well, you can fight and survive.'

EPILOGUE

It's now the middle of January 2013. There's snow on the ground. There's been another hostage crisis, this time in Algeria. The news continues to rumble on and never seems to get any better.

I look back at 2012 with little fondness, but a quiet pride has emerged that whilst we, both our close and our extended family, were facing up to awful health problems, we survived and in fact there were many high points in our year that caused welcome distractions – The Olympics, Sophia and Isabella appearing in a national advert, Sam learning to read and getting so much pleasure from it – oh, and particularly for me, the thrill of watching Andy Murray win his Gold Medal in the Olympics and then going on to win the US Open.

Above all, we've proved what my dear brother-in-law, Ed, said all those many years ago:

"More people live with cancer than die of cancer."

It's now ten years since George was first diagnosed. There have been some extremely anxious times and he has had to endure some harsh treatment, but had he not gone through this he would never have met his grandchildren, or enjoyed holidays in his retirement. We would not have enjoyed such a long, loving, marriage. His life would have been "you work, you die," and who wants to do that!

We've met other, wonderful, patients along the way and we've also met our fair share of self-centred moaners for whom nothing is ever right. That's life! No two people are ever the same.

We're lucky we've got such a close, loving family. We're aware some people have to go through this alone. We know cancer brings with it emotional and financial hardship. But we also know help is available and is given in kindness. It all depends what the cancer patient and their carers choose to accept, because, sadly, again, no two people's lives are the same and you have to make of your own life what you can. That remains everybody's sole responsibility.

But, more than anything, I've learned to appreciate and respect that one, last, great mystery of life:

None of us know exactly when we are going to die.

So, whilst we're alive, even if we are living with cancer, then life remains incredibly precious. As we've proved, it may not be the life you would wish for if you were able to choose, but you can still enjoy many moments in it.

In closing, this would never have been written without the constant and greatly skilled care George has received, particularly from Dr Ajay Kumar, Nephrologist and Dr Amanda Jones, Oncologist.   Both lead wonderful teams at Jersey General Hospital and it is for the continuance of the care they offer to their patients that all profits from the sale of this small book will be donated.   Thank you for buying and reading it.

I wish everyone living with cancer good health and may everyone affected by cancer have many of those rest days that George, my Mum, Bonzo, Bonnie, the dog and I now appreciate so much.

Acknowledgements

My thanks go, as ever, to my trusted readers – Elizabeth (Monty) Lawrence, Gwyn Garfield-Bennett and Judy Smith. This book was a very different project for me and each gave me the encouragement I needed to carry on when I started to doubt it.

Alan Eaton of AEA Design in Jersey sorted out the book cover for me and whilst he was doing it, I – very nearly, but not quite – had great fun trying to persuade him to buy a black dog for his children.

I am so glad Jim Hobby came into my Mum's life after my Dad died. They are wonderful together. I've always worried that I haven't been able to help them more but my cousins and their partners, Terry Oliver and Shirley and Steve High and Penny have kept a close eye on what was happening in Worcestershire for me. Their honest phone calls made being unable to be with my Mum as much as I would have liked just that little bit easier.

Our family and friends have never failed to support us. I'm so grateful we have them.

There are so many medical staff who have helped George over the years I am frightened I will miss out some names, so I will just say thank you to everyone. You have been wonderful. But of course, to Doctor Ajay Kumar and Doctor Amanda Jones, from the bottom of my heart, I simply say "thank you. We could not do it without you."

Nor could we do it without the help of Family Nursing and Home Care in Jersey, particularly Mo; Jersey Hospice, particularly Gail and Cirsty, and the MacMillan Nurses.

And, of course, what would I do without my dear George? He was the hardest one to show the first draft to but, since he read it, he has been my most avid supporter.

Thanks to you all.

George and I both hope this book will bring a little comfort to others like us who also live with cancer.

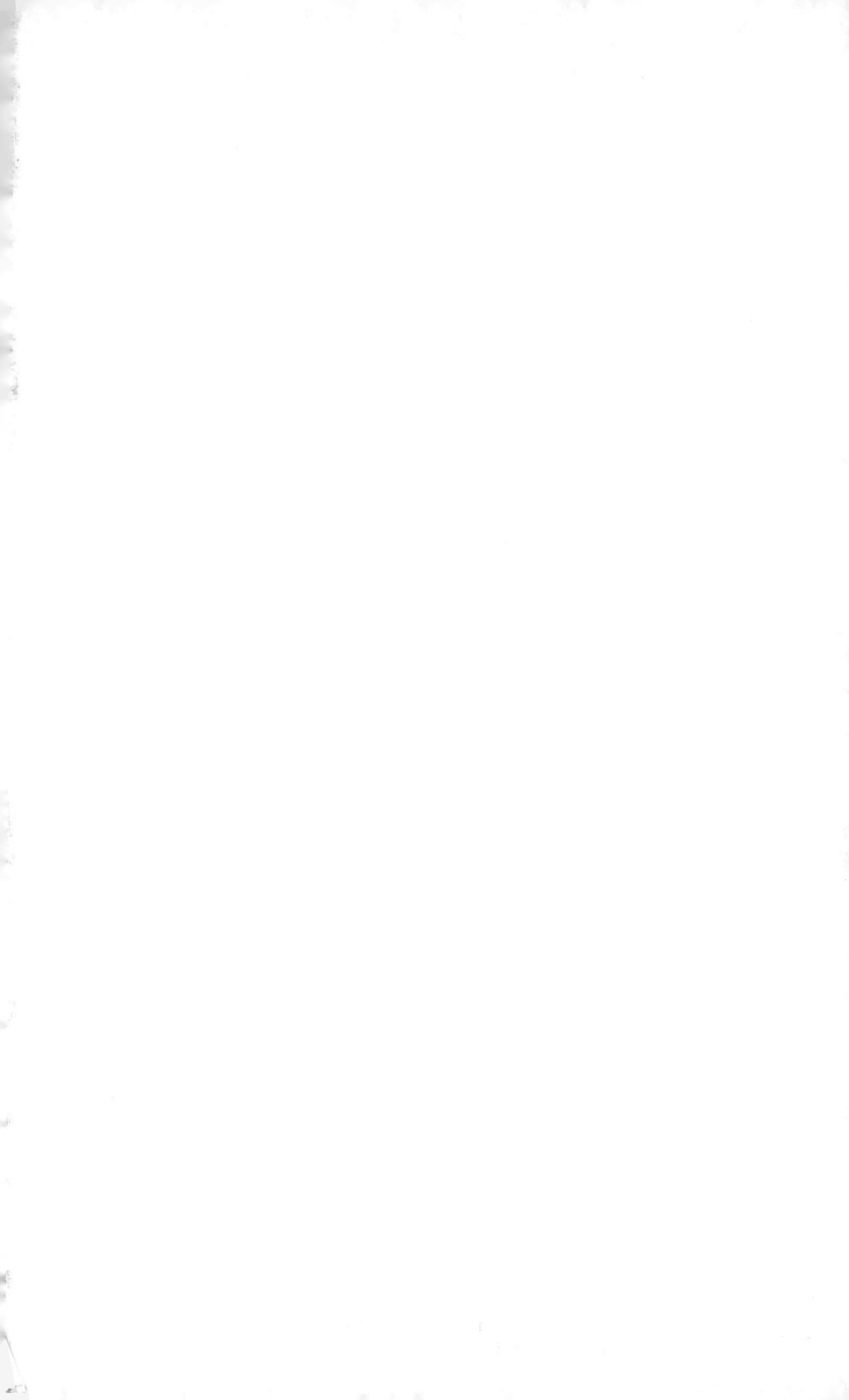

www.ingramcontent.com/pod-product-compliance
Lightning Source LLC
Chambersburg PA
CBHW070551290526
45790CB00002B/646